The Book of Symbiote Diseases

ALSO by PARIS TOSEN

The Man Who Discovered Androids

*World War C: The Secret and Destructive Weather War
between Russia and America*

Captain Starman: Memoirs of a Starcraft Captain

The Book of Stelans

American Androids Critical Edition

Autism & Androids

The Book of Symbiote Diseases

A Radical Healing Approach for Neurodegeneration

PARIS TOSEN

CANADA

Alzheimer's, meningitis, hysteria, Tourette's, seizures (epilepsy), cerebral palsy, narcolepsy, bipolar disorder, schizophrenia, Multiple Sclerosis (MS), autism (ASD), Huntington's, Lupus, AIDS, diabetes, dissociative identity disorder (DID), anorexia, bulimia, depression, obsessive compulsive disorder, cancer, Creutzeldt-Jakob disease (CJD), muscular dystrophy, dementia, Lou Gehrig's, Gerstmann–Sträussler–Scheinker syndrome, porphyria, migraine, Parkinson's.

If there is a cause, there is a cure.

Alzheimer's, meningitis, hysteria, Tourette's, seizures (epilepsy), cerebral palsy, narcolepsy, bipolar disorder, schizophrenia, Multiple Sclerosis (MS), autism (ASD), Huntington's, Lupus, AIDS, diabetes, dissociative identity disorder (DID), anorexia, bulimia, depression, obsessive compulsive disorder, cancer, Creutzeldt-Jakob disease (CJD), muscular dystrophy, dementia, Lou Gehrig's, Gerstmann–Sträussler–Scheinker syndrome, porphyria, migraine, Parkinson's.
Alzheimer's, meningitis, hysteria, Tourette's, seizures (epilepsy), cerebral palsy, narcolepsy, bipolar disorder, schizophrenia, Multiple Sclerosis (MS), autism (ASD), Huntington's, Lupus, AIDS, diabetes, dissociative identity disorder (DID), anorexia, bulimia, depression, obsessive compulsive disorder, cancer, Creutzeldt-Jakob disease (CJD), muscular dystrophy, dementia, Lou Gehrig's, Gerstmann–Sträussler–Scheinker syndrome, porphyria, migraine, Parkinson's.
Alzheimer's, meningitis, hysteria, Tourette's, seizures (epilepsy), cerebral palsy, narcolepsy, bipolar disorder, schizophrenia, Multiple Sclerosis (MS), autism (ASD), Huntington's, Lupus, AIDS, diabetes, dissociative identity disorder (DID), anorexia, bulimia, depression, obsessive compulsive disorder, cancer, Creutzeldt-Jakob disease (CJD), muscular dystrophy, dementia, Lou Gehrig's, Gerstmann–Sträussler–Scheinker syndrome, porphyria, migraine, Parkinson's.
Alzheimer's, meningitis, hysteria, Tourette's, seizures (epilepsy), cerebral palsy, narcolepsy, bipolar disorder, schizophrenia, Multiple Sclerosis (MS), autism (ASD), Huntington's, Lupus, AIDS, diabetes, dissociative identity disorder (DID), anorexia, bulimia, depression, obsessive compulsive disorder, cancer, Creutzeldt-Jakob disease (CJD), muscular dystrophy, dementia, Lou Gehrig's, Gerstmann–Sträussler–Scheinker syndrome, porphyria, migraine, Parkinson's.

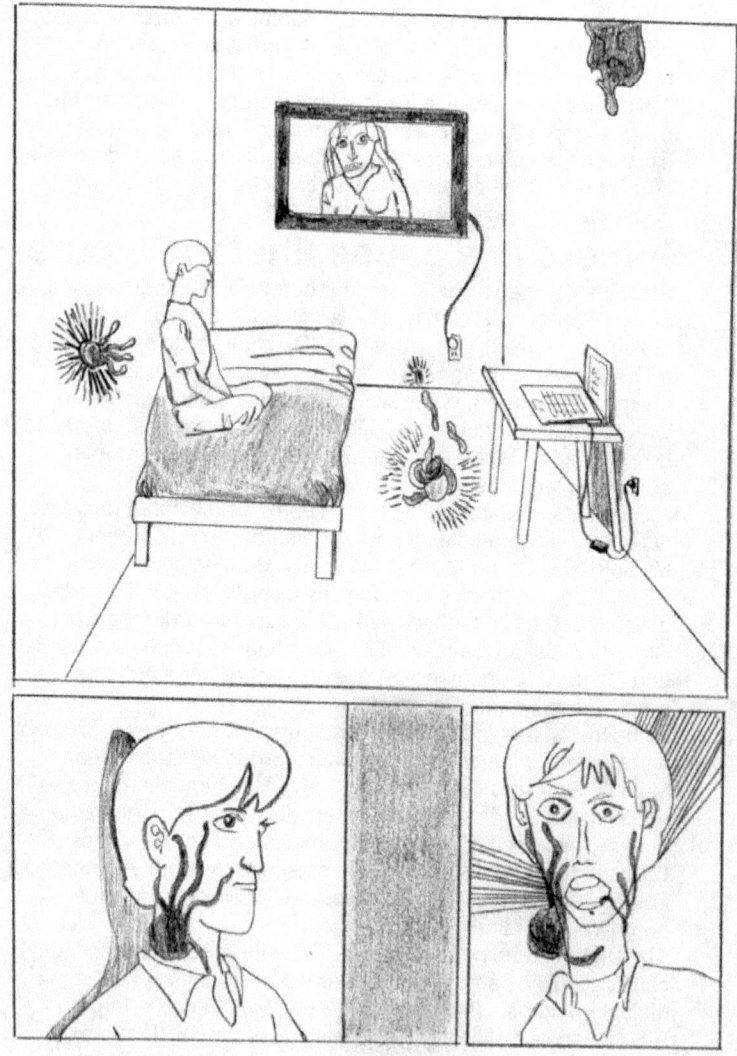

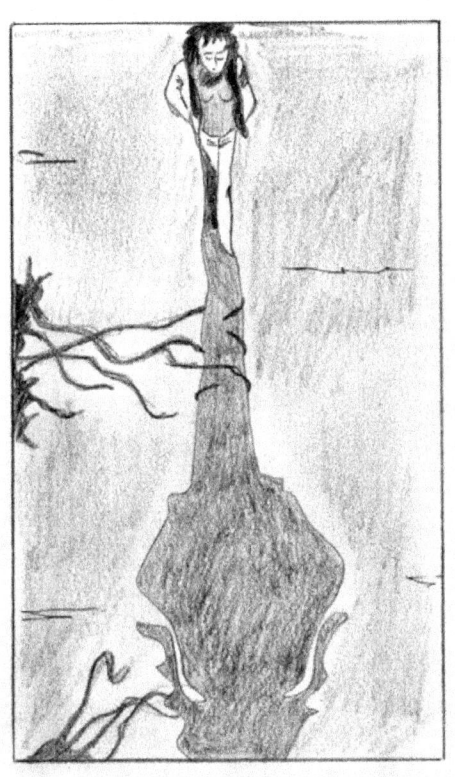

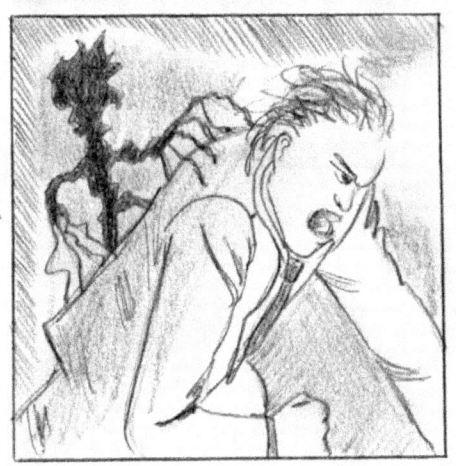

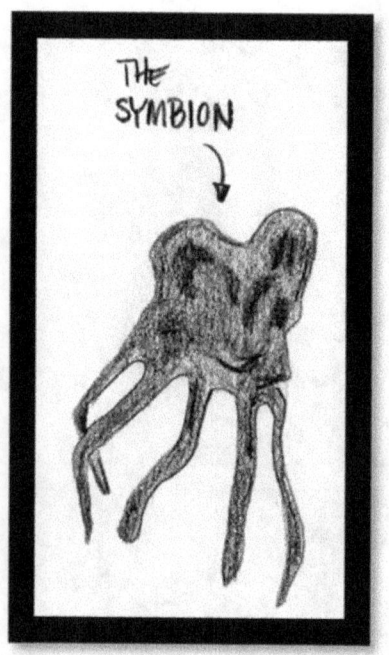

CONTENTS

Disclaimer

This book contains alternative advice relating to health care. It is intended to support orthodox medical advice only. The information contained in this book has not passed scientific scrutiny in any standardized format. The information is largely based on the observations and independent research of the author. The author of this work is not a medical doctor and has had no medical training whatsoever. The publisher and the author disclaim liability for any outcome, medical or nonmedical, that may or may not occur as a result of applying the ideas presented throughout this book. All of the diseases and illnesses discussed herein have been reinterpreted according to the unorthodox laws of reality science. This should not replace the standard definitions of these diseases and illnesses rather to provide a multidimensional medical supplement for a specific demographic of society.

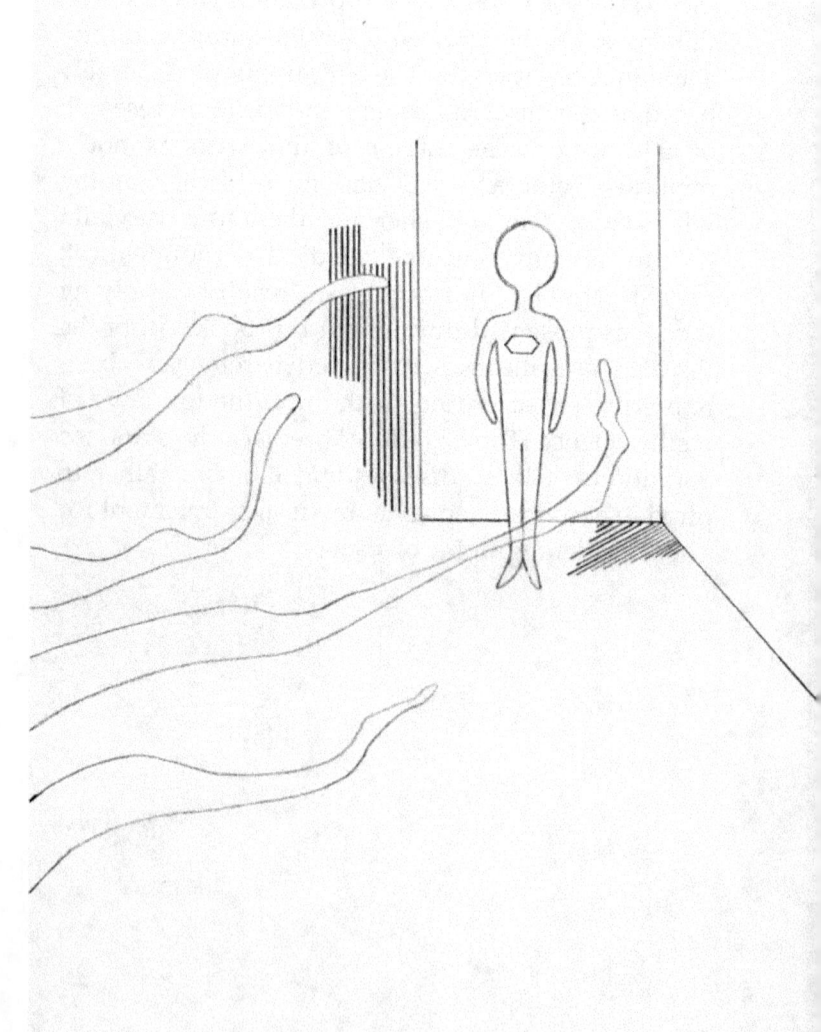

PREFACE

An incurable disease is a chronic illness that has
no identifiable cause and therefore no cure. It is
typically referred to as a degenerative disease
and is sometimes progressive, becoming more
debilitating over time. Parkinson's disease is an
incurable disease. There are 100,000 people in
Canada that will suffer for the remainder of
their lives. Actor Michael J. Fox was diagnosed
with Parkinson's when he was about 30 years
old and has since become a leading advocate of
research in the hopes of finding a cure. That was
twenty years ago.

  Parkinson's was first documented in the early
1800s. It has been around for nearly 200 years,
still without a cure or a cause. Despite the
advances in medicine and technology, the
experts do not know the cause of the disease.
The disease is quite debilitating. People afflicted
with Parkinson's must manage tremors, rigidity,
slowed movements, awkward tics, sleep

difficulties, posture disturbances, and behaviour disorders. Their thoughts are often compromised. Their cognitive speed is slowed, they have poor memory recall, and they have difficulty in executing plans or abstract thinking. Parkinson's sufferers also can experience hallucinations and delusions.

The situation in America is far worse with one million individuals with Parkinson's and estimates of the top 15 nations worldwide suggest that at current growth rates we could see nearly 10 million by the year 2030. There is a neurodegenerative disorder that is crippling people over the age of 65 and as the life expectancy of the individual increases the medical experts have no way to stop it. The blame for this chronic disease is attributed to an ageing population and the lack of corresponding healthcare infrastructure, especially in populous nations such as China and India.

This neurodegenerative disease is focused on the elderly. Ninety-percent of cases are found in people over 65. The mid-brain structure known as the *substantia nigra* is largely to blame and because of its deteriorated state there isn't enough of the neurotransmitter dopamine to maintain all the normal motor movements. And mutated proteins further complicate normal neurological functions. The elderly seem to be in a bad predicament. They must also face dementia and Alzheimer's, two associated illnesses that could lead to premature death. All of them have no known cause or cure: hence, they are incurable.

The elderly are not the only people facing mysterious illnesses. People of all ages can become afflicted with an incurable disease. You have heard of some of them—Huntington's disease, schizophrenia, fibromyalgia, bipolar disorder, depression, Lupus, bulimia, anorexia, Lou Gehrig's, multiple sclerosis, cerebral palsy, dissociative identity disorder, Tourette's, AIDS, diabetes, and autism.

You can't prevent the onset of an incurable disease. It doesn't matter how good your diet is or how much you exercise, or how many sports you play. It doesn't matter how many vitamin supplements you take. It doesn't matter your religious faith. Nor does it matter what kind of career you have or how many charitable donations you have made in your life. If you are unlucky, you will find yourself afflicted with some incurable disease, and if you are a wealthy optimist, you might become a research advocate.

Incurable disease can attack anybody — and this is because the medical experts have not identified the cause. People are prescribed indefinite medication and their families are given a heavy burden for a great many years to come. These diseases have their own will, they happen to good people, they attack talented individuals at the peak of their game, and they come with a list of symptoms that are often overwhelming.

But are they really so mysterious?

The symbiote approach is an entirely new kind of medicine. It is multidimensional healing application. It is unproven and relies on the kind of science that is outside of orthodoxy. I do not think that this *reality medicine* is an alternative medicine. It is a hybrid of advanced neuroscience, genetic regulation, and cosmic energy. During the generalized discussions of a select number of incurable illnesses — since there are far too many to include them all here — I will argue that we have not found a cure because the cause is hidden on a higher dimension. More specifically, the higher dimension is not as nebulas as we might imagine, rather within the electromagnetic spectrum, the difference between the visible and the invisible is a few hundred nanometers.

Whenever we are facing an incurable disease we are ultimately limited by our perception and awareness. Conventional science does not ask unconventional questions. It tries to explain symptoms according to established scientific principles rooted in international research, experimentation, and experience. It assumes that all the best information has been obtained and has been documented.

Reality medicine has nearly nothing to do with the typical understanding of medicine and its reliance on drug applications and conventional treatments; instead this medicine is a technological application that relies on an advanced application of human genetics to manage a range of symptoms caused by multidimensional programs and applications. It assumes that scientific achievement is unfinished. Essentially, it is a first step, a large step, into a world that combines computer architecture with human architecture.

As much as *The Book of Symbiote Diseases* presents and redefines a suite of incurable illnesses and chronic symptoms, it is really a supplement to a greater number of books on the topic of reality science. As well, the efficacy of a symbiote application, just as with any medicine, is intimately connected to the patient; therefore, improving your condition will come about faster by improving your views on the way the world works and by improving your state of mind.

If you are suffering from any of these serious conditions, or similar conditions (since symptoms are often shared), it is imperative that you work closely with your healthcare practitioner and that you maintain any current medical treatment, as necessary. The key is to gradually improve your condition and to gradually reduce your medications, as indicated. A positive frame of mind is, I think, a basic requirement. There is an inverse relationship between positivity and recovery. Your rehabilitation will take on many forms and phases, sometimes improving and sometimes worsening. And the extent of this will largely depend on the length of time the disease has occupied your body.

This book is an entry to an advanced medical approach to neurodegeneration. It has been simplified to a large degree and presented in such a way so as to minimize confusion but many of the concepts here can, and should, be combined with other alternative and unorthodox therapies. I believe that with a continued understanding of symbiotes, we could see the end of neurodegenerative disease in humanity.

If from what I have seen and discovered, both in me and in society, is true then it is highly probable that disease is a construction of multidimensional parasites. It is a difficult concept to convey to a global society that is bent on disease. We have been educated to accept disease as a part of life. As much as we agree with regeneration we still feel that at times we break down and that some people are unlucky in health. Of course the situation on health is not so easily discussed because not everybody knows and wants to take care of their health. Many people don't mind abusing their bodies and will only start paying attention to what they eat after they are overweight or returning from the hospital.

This book isn't about eating right and exercising daily. That is a given. This book focuses on diseases that have no known cause and no cure. These are diseases that destroy lives and families and until now have escaped even the greatest medical minds. The medical community cannot cure what I call the *incurables*. The pharmaceutical companies do not have the drugs in their catalogues to cure the incurables. What remains is a slice of global society, anywhere from 3-5% of a given population, which is forced to live a less-than-full life.

The symbiote hypothesis offers the kind of healing doctrine that identifies the cause of incurables. What does that mean? That means that as long as we have a cause — and if that cause is accurate enough — then we are that much closer to a cure. I think we still need time to cure the incurables and that can come about from medical education. But there is a caveat— the cause I have identified, as you will find throughout this book, is not the kind of scientific convention you would expect. It is a multidimensional convention and that means that in order to fully resolve the issues with incurable disease we have to raise the bar on medicine.

I am raising the bar on medicine and I am doing so from a solid foundation of principles in reality science combined with years of environmental and personal observation. I have been using reality-based healing philosophies to maintain my own state of health under very severe environmental conditions. This is now the tenth year of that process.

It started with the understanding of the synthetic humans, the ones on Capitol Hill. After examining the probable medical mechanisms of androids, specifically the activation of the mid-brain *substantia nigra*, I was led to examine people with Parkinson's disease. I had already been familiar with three other mysterious conditions; schizophrenia, autism, and encephalitis lethargica—all of these were connected to androids and therefore connected to synthetic DNA sequences. I found myself experiencing some of the symptoms listed in these diseases even though I did not have the disease myself. I thought, *well this is strange.* Why do my symptoms seem to come and go if these diseases are so serious, progressive, and debilitating?

Then I realized that I had been battling flu-like symptoms for many years. I had gone through periods of narcolepsy. I had experienced numbness in my limbs, migraines, dry mouth, memory loss, and dealt with mood swings that had no apparent cause. These symptoms were not the result of a bad health or a middle-aged crisis, rather a result from my interaction with advanced multidimensional agents. I had never considered them as medical conditions because I knew their supernatural origins. Plus, I had always been a health-conscious guy, eating right, taking supplements, exercising—these were artificially-induced symptoms as a result of advanced attacks on my health and state of mind. I was certain that the source was external, but I had never thought of my symptoms as having a medical basis. You see, I was thinking supernatural.

That all changed when I began to look at people with Parkinson's and Alzheimer's more closely and I began to notice the evidence of artificial interference. As I explored the symptoms of incurable diseases, having a strong understanding of my work on synthetic humans and my own health challenges, I began to see something really amazing. I began to see that all of these symptoms could be technologically produced. That epiphany led to a discovery — the symptoms of incurable diseases could be artificially-induced when interpreted on a multidimensional level.

Medical experts have never had the opportunity to see the connection between these incurables and synthetic DNA because synthetic DNA had only been discovered in 2010. My android discovery demonstrated that synthetic DNA had been around since at least 1939 because the oldest android, a woman, was born in 1940 and she was synthetic.

I further traced back synthetic human influence to the late 1800s, more than enough time for a worldwide synthetic human demographic. And all of this meant one thing — people afflicted with an incurable illness or disease have some amount of synthetic DNA. These are usually bizarre illnesses with unexplained aches, neurologic and psychiatric disturbances, altered levels of consciousness, pains with no source, attacks without warning, remissions without warning, and drugs without curative effects.

These are very serious diseases and afflictions and to suggest that I have discovered the chief cause can seem arrogant and misguided. But it doesn't change the fact that I think I have discovered the cause to incurables and it is rooted in reality science principles.

This is a new kind of medical doctrine that is perfectly suited to address conditions that conventional medicine has failed to cure. The immediate benefit is the low financial cost. There is no expensive diagnostic machinery or application at this time. In fact, you need only one very advanced piece of software, your genome, and since everyone has a genome everyone has a chance to be cured. The most significant hurdle is the paradigm shift. An identifiable cause will lead us to a long-lasting cure.

The Book of Symbiote Diseases is an introduction to a twenty-first century healing application. I have only myself and my observations to rely on and they have told me that there is a profound healing art that we can tap into. I have had to tap into this medicine in order to stay alive. You, on the other hand, may want to tap into this cosmic medicine to restore your long lost health or to help save the life of a loved one. There is no guarantee of any cure or remission. There never is because all cures are intimately tied to each individual. What is true is that we now have a new *cause* to consider and some new approaches to healing, and within that spectrum of truth I think we are well on our way to making incurable disease a thing of the past.

Paris Tosen

INTRODUCTION

He originally wanted to become an Egyptologist and ended up choosing medicine, but the work of Carl Jung would eventually bring psychoanalysis to the world. Jung, close friends with Sigmund Freud for a period of six years at the start of the twentieth century, straddled the fine line between science and the supernatural. His enemies were quick to brand him as a mystic while he himself insisted that he was a scientist who happened to be studying a field of science that had mystical qualities. In an interview with the BBC in October 1959, John Freeman of *Face to Face* asks him to recount the turning point of his work. Jung, well into his eighties and a couple of years from death, shows a remarkable interest in his clinical memories.

He recounts a "disassociated schizophrenic" patient in one of the clinics, a committed man of 20 years with "no particular education," who asks him to come to the window to look at the sun. The patient, mentally ill in the eye of anyone else, shakes his head left to right and tells an intrigued Jung that if he moved his head in this fashion he would see that the sun is the origin of the wind. At the time Jung thought the man was just crazy. Four years later he happened upon a paper about a newly-deciphered Egyptian papyrus on magic that essentially described how to see the "origin of the wind" from the sun by shaking your head from side to side, turning east to west: the very same technique that the man with chronic schizophrenia had tried to teach him. The magic papyrus had been published years after his encounter with the crazy man.

Jung was a rare intellectual who wholeheartedly held to the idea of Maslow's self-actualization, something he called *individuation,* and his life's work was dedicated to his own self awakening. In the same interview, when asked about the first time he first felt his own individuated consciousness, Jung, pipe slowly pulled from his mouth, leans in responding: "That was in my eleventh year. There I—certainly—on my way to school, I stepped out of a mist. It was just as if I had been in a mist, walking in a mist, and stepped out of it and knew 'I am...I am what I am.' And then I thought, but what have I been before? And then I found that I had been in a mist. Not knowing to differentiate myself from things. I was just one thing, about, among many things."

After Jung and Freud went their separate ways, it was the Swiss psychiatrist who continued his research on the mysterious inner stratum inside each of us. Freud, on the other hand, continued "the talking cure" of Dr. Josef Breuer and used his psychotherapy to remove blocked emotions, memories, and traumas. While his colleague focused on undischarged sexuality, Jung attempted to unify the conscious with the unconscious.

What is appealing of Jung's focus, since I am no expert on Jungian psychology, is not only his willingness to understand schizophrenia but more so his recognition of some internal intelligence. The kind of intelligence that would happen upon my personal research into the multidimensional qualities of each of us, only my discoveries would coincide with artificial intelligence.

The world runs according to human science. The world runs according to human science, and at the same time, the world does not run according to human science. Human science is the result of a human interpretation of how the world is run. The way I see the world is not the way any scientist sees the world. I have been able to read between the lines of logic and lunar satellites. I am a rather simple Canadian man with a degree in international business. I have life experience, as everyone else. That puts me in a very large playing field of average folks. There are many millions of people, younger and older, who are far better educated, with far more talent and with far greater perception. But I have been gifted with a very substantial imagination. I have a Ph.D. in Imagination and this has allowed me to not only survive my encounters with cosmic beings from other dimensions, but it has allowed me to expand my awareness to areas well outside of the best human logic.

I began applying my awareness to extraterrestrials and to reality architecture and it was hard work. They were terrifying times indeed. I saw a great many truths after I realized that this planet is occupied by a nest of nonhuman cultures and that the major governments and their respective secret society offices knew about them. My main work has remained on reality science and the hidden multidimensional architecture that is supporting this field of existence. What is keeping us alive has nothing to do with oxygen and everything to do with existential physics.

My work took a major turn in late 2008 when I discovered the androids on Capitol Hill. I detailed that discovery in my book *American Androids* and created quite a number of books and videos to support my extravagant theories. It took me two years to properly decode what I had seen, plus I had been preoccupied with the evil alien propaganda. When the demand for more information on androids literally took off in January 2011 I was then forced to further decode the androids.

As much as I thought that my discovery was impressive and ground-breaking, and even perhaps that I had reached the pinnacle of my under-classed abilities, I knew in my heart that there was something more yet unspoken. I thought that perhaps I would not need to look into it because we had enough science fiction material to last us all for quite a while. You know how sometimes when a woman becomes pregnant and after about nine months there's this unborn child that wants to come out and it doesn't care what the mother wants? Well, as much as I tried to suppress the birth of my next topic, having not realized I was impregnated, everywhere I looked I was reminded that I could no longer suppress it, that it needed to come out. I would look around to see if any others were discussing it. I thought, if someone else is talking about it, if someone else understands, then I wouldn't have to give birth to this idea.

It isn't easy giving birth. I had done it a few times. Now I am not talking about babies. I am talking about cosmic knowledge and ideas. My last idea, human-looking androids, was very painful and it cost me my life, among other fees. I wasn't ready for the next cosmic child. The more I looked around the more I saw that this topic needed representation and I also saw that no one else had a clue what it was, and no one was even close. Like I said, I have a very sturdy imagination. It doesn't make my domestic life easy, but it does give my alter-ego plenty of things to contemplate.

This new cosmic bundle of joy had to do with reality medicine. I had established some practical concepts in reality science and was comfortable with it, but medicine would be a whole new thing. Yet, every time I studied society, I saw there was an under-represented class of people, diseased people for that matter, who were stuck with no solutions. They had diseases like Huntington's, Parkinson's, Alzheimer's, Lou Gehrig's and a host of many others, even less tragic diseases, yet still painful, like fibromyalgia and diabetes. These diseases all had two things in common. These two things were found in all of these diseases and I remember them clearly from my youth when my father was diagnosed with schizophrenia.

What were these two things? No cure and no known cause.

The best medical doctors in the world did not know what caused the diseases I was studying. Not only that but they did not have a cure. They were baffled. Not baffled enough not to prescribe medication, just baffled enough to say, "We do not have all the answers." The best human science had failed millions of people and millions of families had to cope. And some of these diseases resulted in death.

So here I was, having no medical training whatsoever, looking at these incurable diseases and thinking that this would be my next field of study. The androids weren't enough. I needed something even more impossible, well, why not try incurable diseases? Perfect. What I knew was that these incurable diseases were intimately connected to my android theory and therefore that told me one clear thing—these were synthetic diseases. Since no respectable scientist would ever believe in my wild theories, and likely had never even heard of me, I would be alone on this one.

Then there was one more key — me. I was the third key for I had been attacked by the advanced agents who built the androids and somehow managed to survive. My survival allowed me to see firsthand their technology, a rather impressive thirty-first century technology. One of their technologies used against me would now be used to cure incurable diseases. You can imagine some of the statistical improbabilities that have so far occurred in this discussion. I am an average man with no medical training. I have met extraterrestrial beings. I have seen how reality works, and documented it extensively.

I have discovered genuine living androids in the US government and explained their operations. I have entangled with the android makers, advanced peoples not from this earth, and survived. And now I have seen a missing link with incurable diseases and I think that by applying reality medical concepts to these diseases, diseases that not even the best medical doctor can cure, that I can eventually find a cure. Suffice it to say that if I think rationally, not something I like to do, I would say that this thing is absurd. But I like absurd. Absurd is anything but boring.

This book is about me examining a portfolio of incurable diseases using the observations of symbiote attachments. The symbiote application is a multidimensional medical technology and can provide answers that not even the best medical equipment (eg MRI) can provide. I think the fact that these diseases are incurable points to the fact that they exist in other dimensions and that modern science cannot access those dimensions. I will not present any measurable cures in this book. Any cure will be totally dependent upon the patient's ability to be open-minded.

What I hope to show you here is that some of the most mysterious and debilitating diseases are in fact not what they appear to be. Using reality science principles, I want to show you that there is a new dimension of human interaction and it is in this dimension the true origins of incurable disease. The better we can understand and accept this as a plausible scenario the more likely we will be able to indeed find these people a cure.

If you are diseased or if your family member or friend is suffering from an incurable disease, chiefly the ones I discuss here, then please know that there is something else going on and that we are that much closer to finding a solution, so hang on for now and in the near future we will have something to reduce your pain and suffering. The key is to remain positive for the time being.

What I have discovered over a number of very crucial years is not only that reality is a manufactured environment, but that life is a technology. As difficult as that first step was it was not the final step. It should have been the final step and, indeed, I have been led to believe by all the monks and great gurus (eg the Buddha) that the final step (ie Enlightenment) would be when I saw past the illusory fields of life and into the cosmic architecture of existence. As mindboggling as that will sound to any normal, rational human being, I can say without any hesitation that enlightenment is over-rated and is itself an illusion. Yes, enlightenment is itself an illusion, and it is an illusion that very few individual have made.

I am going to argue throughout this alternative book that these ailments have no cure and no cause in orthodox medicine only. As you move through these chapters you are going to be presented by me, a reality scientist, an unorthodox science, a new interpretation of most of these key ailments. Again, I have no medical training whatsoever. I have studied these diseases both in books and in person and have a solid grasp of the symptoms.

Symbiote observation is based in the core principles of reality science. Since most of you do not know very much about reality science, I will intersperse as much relevant information as possible. I will focus this book on the cause of these painful chronic symptoms. Let us make no mistake, since at times it might not be clear, we are dealing with something that is real. These are very serious diseases and many families have been overwhelmed with them.

Parkinson's disease is not a joke. I may take a light-hearted approach to some of the symptoms for teaching purposes, but I know full well the seriousness of the disease. In fact, as you shall see, I know exactly how serious these things are to human life.

SYNTHETIC NATURE

The best way to explore an entirely new organism is to explain an entirely new science, specifically the science of reality. It is essential that we come to terms with the real qualities of life if we are to properly interpret the case for incurable disease. The real quality of life is not an easy matter and may require a significant amount of time to make proper sense. Starting today is as good as a time as any.

You're not reading this book because you want to look beautiful or because you want to be rich. You are reading this book because you are dealing with some kind of incurable disease with a mysterious set of symptoms. You may have this disease or someone you love may be afflicted. Perhaps you are exploring alternative medicine and you've decided to read up on technological medicine. This is essentially the direction we are headed. It is early in the game yet. Reality medicine is a branch of healthcare that applies advanced understanding to eradicate disease. In our case I have decided to start at the kinds of disease that the best experts in the world cannot cure, the incurables.

An incurable disease cannot be cured because, in my view, it is not a biological disease. I feel obligated to remind you that I am not a medical doctor and have no medical training whatsoever then again the highest paid medical doctors cannot cure the incurable diseases. Oftentimes they do not even know the cause. I think that these diseases can be cured because I think I have discovered the cause — *symbions*.

We'll get more and more into the symbion discussion as we move through each chapter. You will not find every incurable disease covered here, but I think that there are a number of shared characteristics and a similar set of symptoms that you can apply across a broader group. As I began to explore the cause of these incurable diseases, I began to truly see the extent of illnesses that have baffled doctors. Even more important, as you will see, is the historical prevalence of these diseases.

Many of these diseases have been around for centuries, even perhaps thousands of years. How can a particular disease — a set of symptoms — exist for thousands of years even though the human life form has gone through countless genetic mutations? We could argue that the disease mutated along with the human species. Experts will point out that some virus strains may become dormant for centuries and then all of a sudden may attack an unsuspecting organism. For unknown reasons a disease may slip into remission, lying dormant until some critical trigger sends the person to the hospital.

I will argue throughout this exotic book that diseases are artificially-induced and that their appearance is not by the chance as experts would have us believe. The key to understanding all of this rooted in the nature of reality because essentially we exist because of nature. Without nature we could not exist. It is the platform of existence. If the plants do not grow from the dirt and if there isn't enough oxygen in the atmosphere we are dead. If the sun was turned off we would all cease to exist. In fact, the sun is the reason that the plants grow and the reasons why this planet is alive, but life is a funny thing. Everything in nature appears to be alive and moving and growing, but are these things alive?

This is not an existential question. This is not a book on spirituality, although this may be the strongest interpretation. This is an advanced science. According to this science, we live in a synthetically manufactured planet. It has been created using the kinds of technologies that are, say, a billion plus years ahead of human science. If you were to take the super computer and evolve it by a billion years you'd get Nature in a Box. Nature itself is a technology. It is synthetic; a quality so advanced that to our eyes it appears real. It only appears to be real because we have fundamentally forgotten our origins.

If nature is synthetic and we exist because of nature; that is, without nature we would die out then it must be true that we are synthetic. Yes, we appear to be real and biologically gifted, but these appearances are deceiving. It is a deception and it is not by accident. We are deceived by design so as to enjoy the experience of our journey. By removing the technological element we can enjoy the magic of life. But what has happened across the centuries is that we have been completely cut off from our synthetic origins. Instead of remembering them from time to time, we have simply removed them and have allowed other masters to keep them from our knowing.

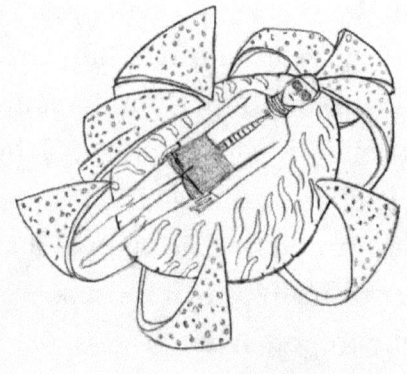

I cannot discuss the cause of disease without discussing the nature of reality. If life is a technology, as I insist, then disease, because it is rooted in life, is also technological, right? If nature is synthetic and the human being is synthetic then disease is synthetic. It must be the case. So in order to properly cure an incurable disease we have to adopt a synthetic mindset. It is a necessity, unfortunately. This may become a bigger hurdle to achieve than understanding the cause.

The human life form is a multidimensional form. It can have multiple meanings and interpretations. For the purpose of this book, I'd like to simplify the human being a little. In doing so, I hope to give those people suffering from a mysterious disease (affliction) a chance to find a way to end the suffering. Because we are technologically-gifted it is the case that each of us is designed from the start with the necessary tools with which to handle the negative aspects of this synthetic environment, but because we have been disconnected for a very long time and likely are functioning at a very low level of performance, the road to recovery will not be immediate. Each of us will require time to heal and to reverse our illnesses, and not everyone will make it. Not every person will have the will and tenacity to make it out of this jungle alive. That should not discourage anyone from trying.

Do not let others discourage you from applying synthetic healthcare.

We can split the human body into two essential bodies. There is the physical body, a synthetic material of bones, flesh, and blood. And then there is the machine body, a multidimensional material that is wholly immaterial. We can say that we have a material body and inside of it we have an immaterial body. It is going to be the immaterial machine body that we need pay close attention to because whatever is done to the immaterial body ripples outward to the material body.

Incurable disease in particular originates from the immaterial body and cannot be cured by tending to the physical body. Again, while it is true we are all made of flesh and blood this flesh and this blood is synthetic material. It is a kind of living technology and it need care and maintenance. At no time should we devalue our existence because it is synthetic. This must be understood by everyone reading this book. Life is of utmost value and importance and we must maintain our lives as a form of dedication to our journey. The journey of life requires a vehicle; hence, the material body. It is true that many people get disillusioned and lost and they turn to self-abuse and addiction.

This is expected. Some minds are weaker than others. If you are stricken with an incurable disease you are required to maintain your health more than normal. You probably are already concerned with a healthy lifestyle, perhaps even mad that you have to face an incurable disease. Why don't people who abuse their bodies get diseased? Why do healthy people get sick?

Part of the reason for this unfairness is due to the fact that the people inhabiting this synthetic planet are not all built equal. In fact, some people are purposely built with exceptional features. But if a person is more advanced than the others and doesn't properly maintain their machine then they are susceptible to not only disharmony, but, more importantly, they are susceptible to an attack.

It is a synthetic world after all and there is more than one human manufacturer and just like what happens in business, competitors get jealous. So there is this other aspect to deal with as well — the more resistant you are to your exceptional features the more likely you will suffer from the attacks of competing manufacturers. Besides, this is not the age to live in ignorance. Humanity has had thousands of years of ignorance and it didn't contribute to evolution all that much.

Now, we have a synthetic environment, a synthetic species and a synthetic manufacturer. We have all the basics to move to the next level. My extensive work on reality and androids (eg *American Android Critical Edition, Reality Science* books) has adequately covered the technologies of existence so it is will not be repeated here. What you have here is a good summary of the situation you are in. You are alive and at the same time you are not alive. You are not alive because you are synthetic and, just as is the case with a laptop computer that means you can never be alive. You are turned on to some extent and you have basic functionality. Again, the only way we are going to break the illusion of life is if we use a more direct approach. It is a very fine art. It isn't perfect.

THE BOOK OF SYMBIOTE DISEASES

This book, like most of my books, will be forthright, smart, and imaginative and this is not suitable for orthodox minds, and it is not suitable for those who are not ready. A person with an incurable disease is in an ideal position to explore this material because they have not only run out of option and money, but because they feel they have nothing to lose. They have lost the fear of new knowledge because their search for answers has become greater than their fear. People who are healthy will not have that same motivation.

You may have a loved one, perhaps a sick child, that is suffering and you may be a person of compassion who is unafraid to explore new ideas. I make no promise of a cure. This book is about the cause of incurable disease and the healing philosophies of reality-based medicine. By the end of this book you will be familiar with the cause of a number of incurable diseases. That cause is synthetic. It is technological and the more able you are to accept the synthetic nature of life the closer you will be to finding a permanent cure.

All of these notions and ideas are based on my direct experience and observation. So, I am not here to give you other people's accounts and the advice of other experts. This knowledge has been carefully extracted from the most baffling and mind-boggling seriousness and is being presented in a simplified format. The nature of life is a profound discussion in itself. It is a divine discussion that we haven't the space for.

Before we jump into incurable diseases and symbion devices, I think it is necessary to introduce a new kind of energy, cosmic electricity.

Cosmic Electricity

You are familiar with electricity. You rely on electricity every day. The home you are in is electrically gifted. The city your home is located is flowing with electricity. You cannot see electricity flowing through the wires. You can measure it with a specific instrument. You can also see its result — the light bulb is lit therefore you know that the power is on. The refrigerator is cold therefore you know that it is receiving electricity and electricity is power.

We are so used to electrical power that we forget just how mysterious it is. Where did electricity come from? It did not come from the sun. It did not come from the tree. Electricity came from science. Scientists built fanciful machines that produced electricity. Each city now comes with one or more power plants and these power stations power the network of buildings including your house or apartment.

Electricity today is a standard of life, but this was not the case of Neanderthal man. Early man did not have electricity; instead their best technology was probably fire. Fire produced everything in the form of heat. Heat energy was used to roast meat. We still use energy for cooking although we have replaced fire with electricity. Many homes use electricity for cooking. The electric stove and the microwave are good examples. Some people prefer the gas stove (or wood burning), but may still rely on an electric tea kettle.

The human body also produces small amounts of electricity, chiefly in the heart and brain. The brain is electrically (and chemically) active. The heartbeat is a result of an electrical pulse. Already we can see our electrical connection to the inventions of our scientists. But now we have to accommodate the immaterial machine, the one I pointed out. The immaterial machine does not run on electricity and that is because electricity is too material. The immaterial machine, the real you, is a very finely tuned device, and it is very sensitive. It only requires a refined energy to keep it alive. Too much or too little energy will cause problems and imbalance. The preferred energy of this immaterial machine is cosmic electricity, something I call *arvicity*.

Arvicity is short for arvic electricity. It is a term I borrowed from a fantasy novel series I wrote, starting with *The Nivian King*. Arvicity is a higher dimensional energy that is present throughout the cosmos, and it is so advanced and refined that we haven't the instrument to properly measure it. Well, that isn't entirely true. We have ourselves. The fact that we appear to be alive is proof positive that arvicity is flowing, like the light bulb. If you have a light in your eyes, you have arvicity flowing through you.

Arvicity is a cosmic form of power. It is very advanced and cannot be accessed by ways of brash ignorance. In fact, the harder you try to access it the more it will escape you. Arvicity is accessed through calmness and introspection. It is the kind of free-energy that this planet desperately needs and has remained elusive, blocked by man's ego.

The immaterial machine runs off of arvicity and arvicity is being fed throughout the reality architecture. Some people, those with a better connection to the high life, will be even more enriched and have greater spiritual power than those who live a more material existence. The more you are able to access this arvic network, like the light bulb and the stove, the more likely you will be able to reverse your incurable situation. Arvicity has a truly amazing regenerative capacity because it is cosmic and fundamentally eternal. It cannot die and therefore if you can gain a better access to it you can experience a more regenerative effect.

You have these two bodies — one of them is a material body that runs on electricity and the second body, the central body, runs on arvicity, cosmic electricity. So if you want to correct an incurable disease, knowing that it originates on the immaterial body, you need to necessarily improve your connection to the arvic networks.

Additionally, as you will see, the cause of these diseases is primarily made of arvicity, at least all abnormal forms of it, and the greater your access to arvicity the greater your ability to deal with this troublesome pathogen. And besides yourself, there are others who can utilize arvicity to put an end to your suffering.

SYMBION ATTACHMENTS

The Nobel-prize winning neuropsychiatrist Eric Kandel once wanted to be a psychoanalyst like his idol Sigmund Freud. Kandel sought to "develop a biological basis of Freud's structural theory of mind." He went on to study the biochemical changes in neurons in regards to memory. His research in short-term and long-term memory furthered the pioneering work on the nervous system by Santiago Ramón y Cajal, Camillo Golgi ,and many others, all of whom he references in his award-winning book, *In Search of Memory: The Emergence of a New Science of Mind.*

Kandel is keen to explain the basics of neuron signalling in the brain. A neuron is composed of three basic parts: nerve cell, axon, and dendrites. The nerve cell is the cell body that contains the nucleus. The axons are wires that transmit signals and the dendrites are the receptive elements.

The axon of one neuron communicates with the dendrites of another neuron at a special region known as a synapse. Neurons are discriminatory. They choose who they want to communicate with just like people who choose certain people to make friends. The neuron is an advanced sending and receiving device and their selection of other nerve cells leads to the formation of neural circuits. These are predictable circuits and not random nets.

Freud succeeded in accessing unconscious memory because he developed a communication protocol that could not be blocked by the ego, and also because of Freud's strong conviction. This was long before the work of Kandel in molecular biology and the properties of human memory.

The symbion pathogen not only can access repressed thoughts and feelings, in addition it affects memory and the electrical signalling of the brain. We already know that nerve cells propagate electricity and are electrically charged with high concentrations of ions and proteins. According to Kandel, based on the work of

Julius Bernstein in 1902, the nerve cell membrane only processes potassium ions.

These positively charged ions create a stable membrane potential as they displace positive-

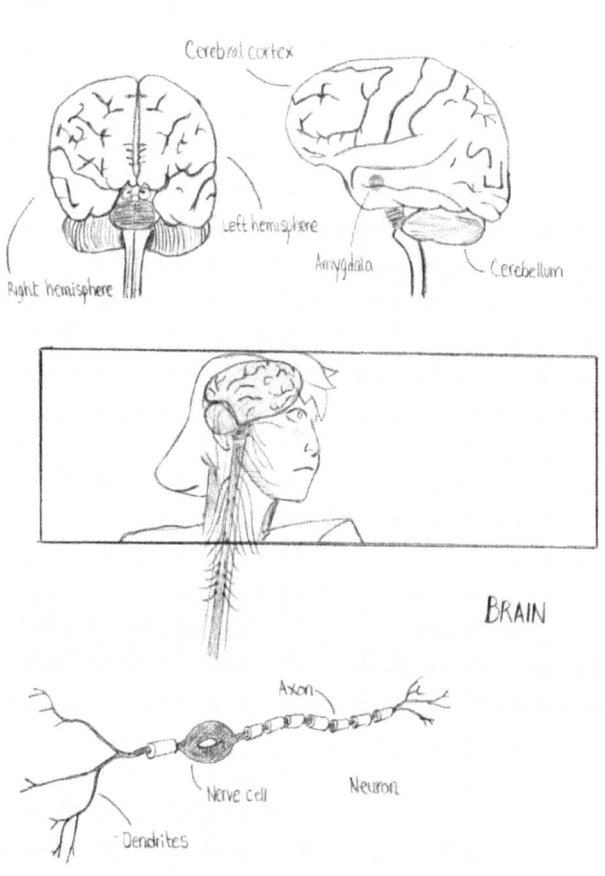

negative charges inside and outside of the cell. Bernstein's membrane hypothesis overcame any supernatural explanation for brain signalling and nervous activity. If the signalling of the nervous system could be explained by science then behaviour could as well.

Brain signalling represents the flow of thoughts, emotions, and memories inside the skull and this could be explained by the action potential in a cell. Just after World War II, the work of Alan Hodgkin and Andrew Huxley led to the ionic hypothesis. They were able to explain how sodium and potassium channels in the neuron generated action potential along the axon. Kandel explains, "Most important, the ionic hypothesis set the stage for exploring the mechanisms of neuronal signalling on the molecular level."

Mental functioning is dependent upon neurons and their ionic exchanges. Proteins in the ion channels that do not function properly or that have been imitated could be responsible for neurological disorder. In our case, an external agency capable of protein mutation would be enough to cause brain-related diseases. Similarly an agency that could cause a mutation in specific genes that code for those proteins would be equally disruptive.

While a symbion pathogen is at first elusive and even supernatural, in fact all it would need to do is to mutate genes or specific proteins and it would be enough to create neurological disease. I will discuss symbions throughout the book in its proper context and this is because it is very advanced and I want to avoid too much misinterpretation. A symbion is a multidimensional symbiote with parasitic characteristics. It is a genomic entity that attaches itself to the immaterial aspects of a host (human) and begins to feed off of molecular exchanges, chiefly in the nervous system. The advantage the symbion has over pharmaceutical drugs and electron microscopes is its multidimensional nature. What does it mean for an organism to be multidimensional?

Just as it requires an electron microscope for a biologist to see a cellular membrane, because the cellular membrane exists on another dimension, a symbion, already rooted in another dimension, can interfere with cellular and genetic processes.

The power of the symbion, besides its invisibility is that it can touch molecular materials and the only real proof we have (so far) is the presence of critical symptoms. By manipulating key chemical processes, things biologists need microscopes to see and study, the symbions can create disorder in the human host. Until now these advanced pathogens have escaped the detection in the scientific community.

As the individual causes thinking to take place, an action that each and every one of us take for granted, and not unlike the ubiquitous mobile phone (smart phone) in our pockets, the nerve cells must integrate both the excitatory and inhibitory synaptic signals in order to ensure a steady flow of information. The intimate neuronal processes and chemical signalling have taken many centuries to understand and has happened to coincide with mobile telephony. In the beginning, nerve cells were believed to utilize only electrical signals and the axons were considered to be like fine electrical wires. The discoveries of electrical nerve signalling would soon give way to chemical signalling after the neurotransmitter acetylcholine was discovered to slow down the heart rate of a frog.

The understanding of the balance of excitatory and inhibitory neurotransmitters in the brain led to the introduction of tranquilizers. These drugs could bind to specific neurotransmitter receptors and alter behaviour. While the majority of synaptic transmission is chemical in nature, there are situations where neurons form electrical synapses.

By the mid-50s, neurologists were content with chemical mediation in the brain, and drug companies were well into R&D. One of the early tranquilizers *Thorazine* (chlorpromazine) was invented in 1950, the first proper antipsychotic. It entered the market by 1953 after tests with psychiatric patients showed improvements in behaviour, it had remarkable effects on reducing chronic psychosis. Shortly thereafter, chlorpromazine was administered to people with schizophrenia and other psychiatric conditions, enough to usher in the deinstitutionalization movement. All of sudden psychiatric hospitals were cleared out as if the magic of Freud swept across North America.

Severe chemical imbalances that once required psychoanalytic treatment now appeared to be treated by drugs. While it was true that the antipsychotics and antidepressants did not produce any real cures, they did save the federal agencies a lot of hospital administration costs. The drawback to these human tranquilizers, apart the side effects, was that some patients had to take them indefinitely. A boon to drug companies, and a new headache to families tending the mentally deranged.

Thorazine was soon enough replaced by an even more stable dopamine inhibitor, haloperidol. It was developed in 1958 in Belgium and would reach the North American market by the late 60s under the *Haldol* brand name. Haldol was 50 times stronger than Thorazine and the drug of choice for treating schizophrenia, people suffering from delusions and hallucinations, the same kind of patients that Jung once studied.

They would be followed with a list of newer drugs with names such as Clozapine, Resperidone, Olanzapine, Aripiprizole, among many others. While the sixties and seventies were about psychotic episodes (excess dopamine) by the nineties people would more likely be suffering from depression (likely from excess serotonin and possibly from not enough serotonin) and it would usher in a new line of drugs called antidepressants. Once again the medical community would be hoodwinked by the technological cause of mental instability.

Throughout my research, I have asked myself as many questions as I could ask. I don't recall all the questions, far too many. Some of the questions included: How is it possible that a symbion can take over a human host so completely? Did the symbions come in several classes — different types of multidimensional organisms — or was there just one class with different programming? How many of these technological pathogens were native to the reality system, how many were created by sorcery (advanced science), and how many originated from the master programmers? My intuition told me that these pathogens were like birds (multiple species present).

My interest in these multidimensional symbiotes only became increasingly evident after I discovered the androids, an accident that changed the course of my life. Although I discovered them in 2008 and 2009, I did not make any sense of my discovery until August 2010. But it wouldn't be until January 2011, nearly six months later when I would see for the first time what was on the table: neurodegenerative disease. In trying in vain to explain how an android functions, using my amateurish neurology I had made attribution to schizophrenia and Parkinson's disease as valid dopamine examples. My father had long-struggled with schizophrenia. But the people with Parkinson's really bothered me. Their suffering bothered me. I did my best at the time to put it aside and to focus on the android specimens.

Another six months later I would see someone else suffering from Parkinson's or Alzheimer's. I knew that I could help but my conscious mind didn't have the education. I didn't even know where to start. But I did know one thing — the symbions were attacking me 24 hours a day. I had been targeted for the past six years and my life had been woefully interrupted. I kept this knowledge private, for personal reasons, but I could now see that these attacks on me were somehow connected to those people suffering from incurables. Again, I did not know how to resolve the gap in logic and at some point I was so moved that I decided I would figure it out: Hence, this impossible book.

What was evident was that the symbions could access long-term memory. When a symbion first attaches to my auric field, almost immediately it is able to activate my neural pathways and to reach into my memories. At first I would recollect my immediate memories and as it attached itself more securely to my nervous system it used my own brain to query deeper memories, even repressed memories. It is not surprising that these negative entities prefer negative memories and I am sympathetic to people who have lived very negative lives for they are at risk of easy takeover.

Symbions prey on negative energy and a person with negative memories is ideal food for these ectoplasmic predators. The stronger the connection to memory the stronger their residency and the more difficult to remove them. I am lucky to have developed an optimistic disposition over the course of my traumatic childhood. Although not perfect by any means, the positive spin prevents any permanent symbionic damage. Positivism is an incredible weapon against these entities, but we have to remember that they are sentient and manipulative, so they will try to convince you to think negative so that they can fully dominate you.

Short-term memory is located in the prefrontal cortex and long-term memory in the hippocampus and cerebral cortex. But the emotional memories, especially those of fear and happiness, are stored in the amygdala. All of these areas are accessible by the symbion's tentacles and they can also be more specific to particular areas for their own selfish purpose. The brain's plasticity provides an amazing defence against an attack, that is if the person knows how to manage their brain's functions, something which most people don't.

Society has never been taught to deal with this kind of threat and neuroscience is still a relatively new field of science. The brain, and consciousness, is still a mystery and given the number of antidepressant and antipsychotic prescriptions we can be certain that not only is society unfamiliar with the brain but medical experts as well. And given the presence and importance of a disease-causing neurological pirate we will need to improve a number of areas if we are to outsmart these invisible cretins.

I have the chemicals to metabolize the necessary proteins to release frozen (dormant) aspects of my memory. So a writer is able to metabolize these memory chains, and the memories of others, as a means of helping society since not all people are equipped chemically. Chemicals can unlock memories but too many memories can overwhelm and too few can make a person ignorant and simple-minded. Symbions use the innate chemical processes to manipulate human memory so as to destabilize the host. If the host is thinking about sexual blunders or family traumas then the host isn't thinking about the present. A prosperous life comes about by focusing on the present and having a good understanding with the past. If you are chained to memories of the past, you effectively live in the past. A society wholly trapped in outdated memories itself becomes outdated and does not develop properly.

The symbion isn't metabolizing memory; instead, they are corrupting neurological processes and neurons and those in turn make the human mind turn inward. A person who recalls a negative experience, playing it over and over again, can fall into severe depression. A person who recalls movies may have delusions and may act out those delusions. They may wish to be more sexually active if they admire a film character who explored that in a famous movie.

The manipulation of memory is a very powerful control mechanism. Activating the wrong memories too easily may overwhelm a person as they are forced to deal with personal issues before they have the emotional scars or preparation to deal with them.

MEMORY ACTIVATION

The prefrontal cortex can consciously access long-term memories. Professor Joseph LeDoux, citing the works of others, writes, "The prefrontal cortex is activated during episodic memory retrieval, and there is also evidence that the prefrontal cortex is involved in the encoding (formation) of episodic memory." This anterior portion of the frontal lobes is an area of the brain that decides how we express ourselves and who we are. What we wish internally is executed through the prefrontal cortex.

A symbionic element (typical or atypical) can activate the circuitry to retrieve working memory and the reassessment of that memory will influence decision-making and behaviour. A symbion can alter the decisions of a person by simply stimulating the working memory. How can this be used in a negative fashion? A recent negative experience, for example a spousal argument or the loss of a valuable job, could be continuously retrieved, even looped, by the prefrontal cortex and the person may not gain the capacity to make new life path choices.

In this sense, it wouldn't take much for an unaware person to focus on a negative experience and to induce unnecessary worry, anger, anxiety and depression. Enough negative emotion and they might seek the help of a doctor or therapist who would likely prescribe medicinal support. It doesn't take much to overcome a mind. According to cognitive psychologists, the mind can only manage about seven items at any given time. If 50% of those items are negatively-swayed then it is probable that the individual in question is no longer thinking straight and is likely seeing the negative.

The prefrontal cortex is particularly interesting because it helps us differentiate between good and bad, and expectation and prediction. We could say that this region of the brain plays a significant role in shaping how you live your life and the longer it is compromised the more likely the person has fallen off the path.

The key is "without awareness" of the symbionic element. A symbion can come in different forms. It can be a worm-like pathogen and it can also be a cloud-like substance, depends on its intended effects and what external agency is involved. When a person engages the invisible cloud-like formation, say at their computer station, the recollection of memories could seem to naturally percolate back into consciousness. For example, the desire to see naked women might be an instant thought at the computer and this fascination may turn into online porn addiction. But this addiction could have an artificial cause, a multidimensional symbion could be suspended so that it engages the prefrontal cortex.

The test would be to see if the clearing up of the computer station, table, chair, and all, on a daily basis, if it would reduce the desire to search for online porn. And as well, since symbions migrate to their hosts, for the person to become more aware of strange thoughts and emotions as symbions try to re-engage their host. With a little effort, it could be demonstrated, as I have done on my own, that a fixation could be reduced and removed by reducing and removing symbionic elements.

It is not a onetime thing. In order to ensure a long-term reunion the person would need to also change their lifestyle and way of thinking, or have a caretaker there to minimize the effects. A person with a severe illness or severely impaired would likely be unable to resolve this highly advanced situation alone. In some cases there may be so many symbion clouds present in an apartment (or home) that a person may not want to leave the apartment. They may stay inside for days and weeks at a time afraid to go outside.

If this is the case it is imperative that this person schedule at least one walk a day, preferably two hours or so at a park or beach. If the weather conditions are severe two one hour walks are just as well. Even a trip to the mall or coffee shop can prove invaluable to the overall mental health of the person. Sometimes these people at home may also have substance issues and other addictions. Ideally people should find time to go outside each day and to interact with the world. When drugs, sex, or other fixations prevent life's normal activities then symbions may be involved, and if symbions are involved they need to be addressed before the human life is compromised.

There is good reason for a writer to sit at home for three days while finishing a novel, but the reasons for watching online porn for three days are never good enough. Blaming these external agencies is also not the path to take to regain the authority over you. The key is to realize that an advanced sentient organism is interested in your vital essence and that you should not allow it (them) to have dominion over you. Your willpower needs to be stronger than it is. Because they can know your thoughts, symbions will often weaken counter efforts by inducing guilt and other negative emotion (eg fear, anxiety). Remember that it shares your executive mind (prefrontal cortex) and has good access to your memories.

On a technical level, it essentially knows you better than you know you. If you try to raise your willpower it will wait to destroy your effort. It will recall all the times you failed. It will drum up memories of abuse or times you made mistakes. It will have you focus on your imperfections and why nobody loves you. But it will do so because it needs you to survive. The symbion is a leech. It is a *vampiric* being.

If you regain control it loses the joyride. It becomes weak and will fade away without another host. So in the presence of regaining your life or overcoming an addiction, there is this psychological and emotional struggle and it can be overwhelming as the tentacles of the symbion are slowly yanked out. The length of this recovery can indicate just how long the symbions have been there. If you do manage to overcome them then be aware that they want to come back as soon as possible so you must not let down your guard. Find health supplements (or learn exercises and techniques to do the same) to boost your immune system and rebuild your life with more positivism, compassion, and general self-respect.

The data in your active memory activates other aspects of your mind and determines what you pay attention to for the time being. Your brain's focus is largely dependent upon what is in your active memory. Your active memory determines what course of action you might take. Many of our essential thinking processes, and even forms of reasoning, are deeply connected to our memory operations. Any agency that can interfere or influence those executive memory functions can therefore alter decisions and courses of action.

It is hard to make sense of your life, and of who you are, if your acquisition of memory is inoperative. In fact, chronic disengagement to long-term memory storage can make a person live a life completely disconnected from who they are. While some people may prefer to avoid old memories, especially traumatic ones, what is true is that facing ourselves, "warts & all," is an essential task if we are to fully know ourselves. The symbion pathogens have no intention of seeing you know who you are for that would not allow them to remain fully hooked into your nervous system so they will typically flood you with negative memories to weaken you or they might also disconnect your mind to long-term memories so that you exist based on a limited self-knowledge and specific memories they themselves control.

They might call upon memories that made you feel worthless so that you continue working as a prostitute (thief, homeless person, investment banker, molester) or that you remain in an abusive relationship. The sentient predator does not care about your life situation. It is not in their concern. They care only to survive and their survival translates into your substandard chaotic life. They feed on neurochemicals and drug addicts, depressed people, and criminals all have an abundance of neurotransmitters upon which to feed.

Even people drive to succeed and in high stakes real estate, entertainment, or industrial business dealings could be susceptible to symbion attachments. Where neurochemicals are abundant, they'll be there. Stable and harmonious personalities do not produce the quantity of neurotransmitters required to keep a symbion satiated. While there is nothing unusual about extreme activity, it is when activities are dangerous or there is a significant shift in personality that it is suspect.

HIJACKING GENES

"High performance computing is now one of the absolute essentials now of biology. Without the biggest computers in the world we can't do what we're doing," says J. Craig Venter, a genomic pioneer dressed in a jacket with jeans, to Richard Dawkins. They are in the midst of a 2009 interview for the Channel 4 UK TV program *The Genius of Charles Darwin* at Venter's high-tech DNA sequencing lab. They walk along the aisles created by rows of these powerful gene machines. Dawkins is a scientist himself, an atheistic evolutionary biologist who penned the book *The God Delusion* in 2006. The book argued that a supernatural creator is a false belief, an argument that sold over 2 million books.

Venter is not afraid to upgrade his technology. The hundreds of DNA sequencers were in the process of being replaced by a single sequencer. What are they sequencing? The genome. The genome is a book of life with 3.3 billion of letters of code. In each of the roughly 100 trillion cells in the human body there are two full copies of the genome. International scientists first attempted to sequence the human genome in 1990 when the Human Genome Project (HGP) was launched. Planned as a 15-year initiative, the HGP floundered and by 1998 only about 3% of the genome had been sequenced. It was at that time that Venter and his team entered the game. With only $300 million, 10% of the federally-sponsored HGP, Venter provided a rough sequence of the human genome in less than a year.

"But, so, sequencing genomes is equivalent at Moore's Law at least which is doubling every one and a half years," Venter is agreeing to Dawkins in the background, "which means that in 50 years everybody can have their genome done in a doctor's office... uh...," Dawkins trying to estimate people's genetic future from his discussion with the inventor of the first synthetic cell. Venter responds, "I'm hoping we get to that point in 5 years."

"In five years!" Dawkins exclaims.
"Yeah, in five years it should be down to
$1,000 which is pretty amazing—"
"$1,000 to have your genome done—
which means that the doctor will
prescribe not a generic cure for what
you've got, but a specific cure for
anybody of your genome."
"Exactly," agrees Venter.

The cost, at the time, of sequencing a genome
was one million dollars. That was down from
$10 million nine years prior. And that was
expected to reach an affordable thousand by
2014, a kind of democratization of the genome.
Venter, head of Synthetic Genomics, was
instrumental in mapping the first human
genome in 2000 (and subsequent years as
sequencing technologies improved), even using
his own DNA as one of the five initial samples.
His follow up performance took place in May
2010 and involved the creation of the first
synthetic organism using man-made DNA
designed in a computer. In a June 2011
interview, when asked on the television news

magazine *60 Minutes* about the shared similarities with reprogramming software, Venter responded, "DNA is the software of life. There is no question about it. And that's key to evolution of life on this planet. And now the key to the future of life on this planet is understanding how to write that software." If only Venter realized that a multi-cellular synthetic organism, aka *human*, had already been invented as early as at least 1939 (reference to the oldest android discovery on Capitol Hill).

While every gene of the genome is in every cell of the body, it is also true that each cell type turns on only the genes it needs. Only certain genes are expressed, the rest are shut off or repressed and this gives each cell its own protein mix to perform its biological functions. Kandel says, "Genes are switched on and off as needed to achieve optimal functioning of the cell." Why are genes important to our discussion on incurable disease? Because there is a genetic basis for antibody diversity.

As early as the 1970s, scientists have realized that the immunological response to antigens is regulated by the expression of genes. Some genes are expressed at certain times and some can be turned on and off as a response to signals coming from inside the body or from the environment. Effector genes, for example, encode proteins to achieve specific cellular functions and regular genes encode proteins that switch effector genes on and off. The process of gene regulation is intimately tied to environmental cues.

If we know from science that gene function is regulated up and down as a response to environmental stimuli, and we are now aware of a multidimensional pathogen, we can now infer that a symbion can influence and alter gene expression. And it can do so invisibly. The human genome can be genetically regulated by a technological device that is beyond the detection of the best scientific machines. The proof that there is some kind of unknown agency at work is the presence of incurable diseases and a whole host of physical symptoms: loss of motor skill, learning disabilities, anxiety disorders, addictions, seizures, hysteria, forgetfulness, and pneumonia.

The neural circuitry is where the human cockpit is located. The release of specific neurochemicals can lead to the activation of genes and the creation of new proteins. A symbion's primary task is to hijack the human cockpit because it instinctively knows that this is the center of gene regulation — control the neurochemical flows and the body can be controlled. For example, a single pulse of the neurotransmitter serotonin increases action at the synapse. When there are repeated pulses of serotonin it causes protein to enter the nucleus where it activates genes. That process could allow a short-term memory to become a long-term memory.

A symbion only needs to block the production of a regulatory protein and if blocked then long-term synaptic change is blocked. So this technological pathogen can gain access to human memory simply by interrupting or activating the creation of the right protein in brain cells.

Not only is the external environment influencing the release of serotonin and the production of protein, but also there is an advanced pathogen inside of the nervous system that can interfere with those essential neurological processes. What is remarkable about human memory is that it can influence human emotions and the expression of human emotions releases neurochemicals. The release of those neurochemicals led to the expression and suppression of human genes. The genes in turn encode new proteins to regulate the body. Having access to human memory is a powerful way to control a human being. The molecular biology of mental processes can be used to a great extent to cause harm to an individual life form and it is orchestrated by advanced agencies that want to cause harm.

The native system orchestrates life as we know it by way of energy flows. Due to multiple classes of inhabitants, interdependent on genetic disposition and activation, there are some people who can intercept these energies, even attract them, and these sorts of people would be the usual candidates for mental illness.

Mental illness, at the same time, isn't contagious. It has long been considered an organic and inherited disease that has no permanent cure. Doctors working inside of a mental hospital may suffer from stress and overwork issues, but they are unlikely to develop schizophrenia. If the reality system is at least partially ordered by energetic wave mechanisms then while a normal class of inhabitants would simply comply or resist a command, a synthetic class inhabitant would be able to interact, even inhabit, this energy.

But there is a problem — human science and psychology has been woefully suppressed and has yet to accommodate these multidimensional energies. Therefore even a synthetic class inhabitant cannot make sense of this energy and can be overcome. This situation likely results with a stay in a mental hospital and/or a treatment of antipsychotic medicines. As well, it is noted, a misguided interaction with these primordial (native) waves of orchestrating energies can lead to incurable diseases. If so, it must be because the human genetic proficiency is too amateur to escape any misprocessing.

A person with limited cooking ability given a professionally-equipped kitchen and a complete list of food items will never be able to achieve the quality of a master chef. The master chef can only produce an exquisite dish, or set of dishes, because of many years of training and practice. Where humanity has fallen terribly short, and has been continued to justify this closed-minded approach—is in the field of multidimensional training and development, areas still disregarded by conventional science. We know these areas as paranormal, extraterrestrial, and supernatural.

Had we acknowledged the value of multidimensional entanglements (eg ghosts, astrology, UFOs), and given the respect they deserve, we would have abolished mental hospitals early on and we would have been able to leapfrog the administration of lobotomies (psychosurgery) and neural tranquilizers. We may have been able to enter the outskirts of energy-based medicine, part of which is utilized in reality medicine.

These opinions are rooted in my own personal observations and should not be treated as a silver bullet to all disease-related problems. My radical healing doctrine has so far a limited application and is chiefly applied to a small set of incurable diseases, some more serious than others. But these diseases are diverse — from schizophrenia to MS, even including diabetes and peptic ulcers.

The medical principles developed so far is wholly-rooted in the symbion pathogen, in its basic form. The extent that the symbion has hijacked the human host, including cultural attachment areas and length of incubation, can inform us as to what kind of cure may be possible. You see, we haven't yet established any proper cure. We have identified an entirely new cause.

The synthetic class inhabitant, although estimated to be genetically augmented, is not necessarily a superior person in the classic sense. And if these synthetics are routinely subject to either psychotic episodes (eg dementia praecox) or to neurodegenerative disease then they are a species at constant risk of extinction. Quite often the result of a lifetime of adrenaline-fuelled episodes, likely punctuated with addictive substances, both in modern times and even say 100 years ago, is hospitalization, drug treatment, and homelessness followed by an early death.

A hijacked body thrust into extremes, lacking the necessary stability of a normal life, improperly nourished and eventually abandoned even by a close knit family will not live very long. In some ways the mental asylum has been replaced by rehab centers, especially in North America. Celebrities falling off the wagon or suffering from a chronic addiction (eg sex) have since popularized rehabs, but rehabs appear to be more humanistic treatment centers.

What remains present is the fact that a class of humans, synthetics, is at risk of a symbion attachment and therefore their livelihood is at risk. Medicating them does not resolve the fundamental cause — a technological possession. Rehab centers have only multiplied as even the patients (guests) learn ways to overcome (or outsmart) the therapy. And why they want to outsmart the therapy (to break the rules) has nothing to do with the good-willed person inside; instead, it is because of a sentient symbiotic predator that is able to overtake the nervous system. Once comfortably in control of the host's nervous system the symbion has control of the host's mind. And because it is symbiotic the host cannot distinguish whether the internal operating system or the external agency is in charge.

In typical fashion, and from the help of treatment experts, it is decided that the addictive substance has taken over the host. Quite often a person under the influence acts and behaves irrationally because of the substance. The drug has taken over. While this is a useful description, because it separates the natural host from a foreign agency, I will argue that the drug is just one of the cravings of the all-together advanced pathogen. Yes, the host is not in charge when under severe addiction, but neither is it the drug. It is the symbion. The symbion is having a joyride and will continue to take joyrides from this highly unusual class of people under medicine can catch up to this technological threat.

We could cure addiction if we could teach caregivers and treatment specialists how to handle symbion pathogens. And then we could teach addicts (drug, alcohol, sex, prostitution, gambling, masturbation, food, violence, crime, lying, pedophilia, laziness, conspiracy) how to recognize when they have been targeted. At this point it doesn't matter all the reasons for their attachment, but it is imperative to reduce their effects. As long as antipsychotics, tranquilizers, therapists, and rehabs remain in abundance we can be certain that symbionic pathogens are feeding on neurochemicals and they have no intention of ever going on a hunger strike.

SYNTHETIC HUMANS

The 22-year old Bertha Pappenheim suffered from hysteria. The symptoms of hysteria in 1880, as documented by her physician Dr. Josef Breuer, included childish behaviour, severe mood swings from high spirits to suicidal urges, and even hallucinations of black snakes crawling along the floor. But that is just a sampling of a bewildering mass of symptoms. Patients with hysteria experienced partial paralysis of limbs, disturbances of vision, crushing feeling in the chest, and seeing a frightening image of an angry male face. The affluent Dr. Breuer noted how Bertha was a brilliant, creative, and strong-willed individual and yet she was experiencing altered states of consciousness.

Breuer was Freud's earliest mentor. Bertha commented that his "talking cure" seemed to have some effect on her condition but it would be several years before Bertha became normalized. Following Breuer, Freud developed his treatments in psychoanalysis and became increasingly focused on blocked emotions and memories. It appeared that the onset of hysteria coincided with a traumatic event in the patient's life. Freud attributed hysteria to undischarged sexuality and why his psychotherapy was focused on releasing the patient's repressed sexual urges.

A death or trauma in the family seemed to weaken the patient severely. The family we know is intimately intertwined and in equilibrium like a series of networked computing devices. When a computer goes offline (death) the network is partially down. When two people die then the network is gone. It is likely the case that a family network is required for a certain period of time before an individual can be self-reliant. Women in the late 1800s were not independent and required family and a male figure.

Women with hysteria tended to have been sexually molested and even had an unexpressed sexual desire. The sexual energy channels open up when a person is genetically activated. The sexual channels are key mechanisms connected to the immaterial machine and sexual identity plays a central role in communication between immaterial machine and material body. When the symbion distorts the sexual energy flows the patient can be distorted. On a psychoanalytical level, as Freud and Breuer observed, sexuality was significant to the hysterical symptoms. The theory of sexuality was not central as the cause though Freud seemed to have focused on sexuality more than others. Usually hysteria was brought on by traumas and deaths.

It is interesting that even in my work and my association with exceptional people, individuals who have incarnated for a higher purpose, there is this theme of trauma. My personal work on trauma and dysfunction of family had identified severe psychic and memory blocks and insisting those traumas were necessary in order to gain access to other aspects of my genetic information. Memory was intimately tied to genetic activation, perhaps a complex terminology, and traumas wreaked havoc on memory systems; therefore, genetic activation was compromised. The loss of specific genes led to the inability, due to unavailable meridians of energy, to handle a symbionic interference.

Symbions effectively jam electromagnetic and neurochemical signals in the body and this jamming causes a whole host of symptoms to appear. This is why I found that the removal, or reduction, of a symbion simultaneously reduced or removed symptoms, without the need for drugs.

The death and loss of early hysteria patient's lives very likely compromised their network integrity. We can infer by genetic design that a family has a similar cluster of existential vibration. That the DNA of each member is able to resonate with each of the other members. This is important for survival and the growth of children. So that when a parent dies the network is temporarily down.

Similarly when a father molests a daughter the daughter's connection to the father's DNA gets corrupted and she becomes ill or depressed. (It must be noted that the symptoms of illness are valid and real, but, at the same time it is important, if not vital, in the establishment of a cure that we upgrade and translate these symptoms using a technological doctrine; otherwise, the cure will never be invented.)

Freud distinguished two states: conscious and unconscious. The fracture between the two created various psychological illnesses. Breuer's approach was to use the cathartic technique as a means of expressing repressed thoughts and feelings, what his patient Bertha referred to as "the talking cure." Freud's approach was less sympathetic as it was surgical. Psychotherapy was meant to penetrate into the memory reserves of the patient in a more forceful manner. Psychotherapist and Freudian biographer Louis Breger writes, "Freud, in contrast, became increasingly convinced of the correctness of his theories and was insistent that when patients did not confirm his view of things, it was their resistance; it was proof that he was right."

Freud's psychoanalytical method involved a brief therapy and a cure, a cure that would not last. Neither did Breuer's more lengthy cures last. A patient's recovery required a number of years even following any treatment.

The rejection by a friend, a group or a loved one, a break-up, on a technological level is not equal to the psychological fallout. When an electromagnetic contact is disengaged from another device there is this phase of signal loss. The accompanying wavelengths that now surround the wiring are chaotic and energetic. When a vehicle changes lanes there is a brief interruption in the equilibrium, the vehicle sways left and right, the occupants feel the strain of their seat belt, and there is a loss or gain of land speed. There may be even a shift in terrain before the new lane is acquired and the vehicle is stable once again. At the human equivalency, the break in a network — death, divorce, fallout, job loss — causes a host of psychological symptoms that not only require psychological therapy, but, as well, exposes the individual to forces in other dimensions, low frequency entities that are attracted to human suffering.

The symbions are able to access the human host better when the host has been psychologically devastated. When there is a loss or a divorce there is an opportunity for a symbion to attack more profoundly than usual. At these low points, oftentimes, there is a sexual shift—a straight woman begins a lesbian relationship, for example, as long as the woman is resonating a steady frequency in a solid relationship or even in continuous relationships then she is much less susceptible to a symbion attack. It is not the case that a woman or man will become homosexual as a result. Homosexuality is only one of many options within the symbion's tool belt.

Multidimensional pathogenic gender influence from a symbion is not the singular reason for homosexuality. There are many reasons for gender preferences. What I have experienced directly, in addition to close environmental observation, is that the homosexual community has been artificially grown, influenced, and shaped by a host of symbion types and is larger than it should be. While this is hard to prove, since we do not have any accurate homosexual population standards and neither do we have the instruments to measure symbions, I can only rely on my observations and personal experience. I have been attacked by these devices and they have worked hard to either flip my gender preference from straight to gay, and failing that they attempted to confuse my gender and to push me into bisexuality.

I remained heterosexual only from understanding myself and learning how to diffuse these entities, but I learned that many of these entities could easily overwhelm an unsuspecting target who would wake up one day gay and because of the neurological reprogramming they will believe that they were always gay. The symbions will have effectively rewired their brain circuitry and memories in order to ensure that the newly-turned homosexual cannot switch back and will remain fixated on their new gender long enough to further strengthen those neural circuits.

I have nothing against gay people per se, but I am fully aware of advanced technologies being used to artificially make people gay and that means not all gay people are supposed to be gay. Based on my work, I would estimate, roughly, that up to 30% of the homosexual community has been manipulated to be gay. This also ties into the sexual energy channels of a person, as discussed throughout this book, because control of the sexual identity is control of the person.

Had a person incarnated for a divine purpose as a man and then during their sexual awakening they were converted to a gay man then the original divine path will have been interrupted because the divine path was fixed on the original gender. It is like buying a car with an 8-cylinder engine and then a mechanic reprogramming the onboard computer to use only 4-cylinders so that you save gas while driving. Sure, the vehicle is more economical to drive, but at the same time it is equipped with the horsepower of 8-cylinders that will never be used.

This does not prevent the gay man from contributing to the planet and society, rather it means that their original life path as decided before incarnation (again, something that is nearly impossible to prove conclusively) has been changed. And this would only benefit the masters of this plane for it alleviates any angelic threats that may have been sent here. This is why it is a very important topic and why I presented it here.

We are not talking about tolerance and human rights, we are talking about divine paths and purpose because they are tied to the material body of incarnation and that is connected to sexual identity because sexual identity determines the wiring in the brain and wiring in the brain determines your genetic disposition and that determines your connection to this false reality.

This will not be relevant to every gay person. In fact, most gay people will live accordingly. You can see by my work that I am focused on a very small percentage of society and that I talk about synthetic DNA and incurable diseases so you can see that my concern is when the life path of special individuals are compromised. Whether they are given some incurable disease or their gender is converted, in either case their life paths have been compromised. Don't let your life path be compromised. The better you know yourself the less likely they can interfere with your life as they have done to me and many others. You don't gain anything by becoming gay and you don't lose anything by remaining straight.

Recall as well that the symbion does not care about making someone homosexual unless these entities were *programmed* to do so. I have seen this to be the case where symbions were created to switch or confuse a person's gender, in the usual kind of symbion attack; the multidimensional pathogen is simply designed to compromise the host so that it can control it for a period of time.

As it access unconscious memory it may discover by accident repressed sexual desires in which case it will feed. But if it accesses deep-seated rage it will feed on that instead making the host full of anger issues and even prone to violence when under duress. And a number of these repressed emotions may surface on some individuals who have avoided self development. People with a higher self awareness and level of independence are able to avoid any real psychological crash and therefore immune to many of the symbion's charms.

Freud's evolution of the unconscious and of storage of repressed feelings became the Id after the book *The Ego and the Id* was published. The Id was a Latinized form of the "It" and the Id represented an ancient energy reservoir. If the Id could not express itself directly then it would direct itself through the ego. Symbions have a remarkable ability to rupture the Id and to infect it with distaste for goodness.

In its place the symbion is able to modify the memory acquisition and to make it negative or positive. While its preference is negativism and repressed desires (eg homosexual urges, need for violence, addictive substances), symbions can also draw forth dreams of a positive nature. In each case the symbion device can not only attract a particular memory or set of memories, more so, it can magnify them.

The magnification of the deep-seated memory can overwhelm and distort the mental processes of the individual. A bad memory can lead to depression. A painful experience can send a man into bouts of rage. An unmet dream can make a person live out that dream even though that dream was better left as a dream. My observations on this tell me that whatever comes as a result of symbionic influence is unnatural and is unrelated to the journey of the person.

People are complicated. They go through many stages of life and they have to deal with many experiences; negative, positive, and mysterious. Depending when a symbion attachment takes place it can have any number of consequences. A person may recover from a childhood trauma one year and then, years later, they may deal with issues with homosexuality.

The host that enters a diseased state is the kind of host that is able to resist the effects of simple symbions, and, in doing so, they evolve at an intrusive level. That intrinsic quality seems to be invariably connected to the genome. There is a remarkable aspect to a symbion target and it has to do with DNA sequences. These technological pathogens seem to prefer people with a particular genetic disposition. Following my work on androids and manufactured realities I cannot help but associate the synthetic identifier with individuals under symbion attack.

On one level it makes sense that a technological device is attracted to a synthetic person or to a person who has at least some synthetic DNA. Synthetic DNA is only a very recent discovery in human sciences, invented in 2010 under Venter's leadership. His team of geneticists created the first synthetic cell "using four bottles of chemicals." The bacterium they created was designed inside of a computer. In my view, Venter proved something very significant: biology is an illusion. When a computer could create a DNA-based organism using manmade chemicals it fundamentally changed the definition of life.

Integral to the presence of these largely invisible pathogens is the redefinition of at least some human beings. It would appear that some human beings have either been synthetically created or have within their genomes a sizable portion of synthetic DNA. And because of this they are ideal victims of the technological predators.

Symbions will at first attack in a milder form, aches and pains, distorted thoughts, memory lapses, and then progress into psychological disturbance. If that is not enough to stop the person then they will bring forth the onset of some mysterious disease without a cause. They are the cause. What has to be true in the case of incurable diseases is that these afflicted people have a strong synthetic quality to their makeup. Perhaps people with weaker genes simply die off from a heart attack or strange accident.

What I have observed in myself is that the more I unlocked my genetic potential, the more I thought about the unthinkable, the more I increased my awareness of the unknown then the more disease symptoms I had to deal with. Had I succumbed to bipolar disorder or depression I would've have the symptoms of MS or even Parkinson's. I was never concerned with the presence of symptoms, as would a normal person.

Plus, I felt that my meditative exercises could alleviate my symptoms and therefore they did not seem permanent. Critical to my survival was a positive mental outlook. Had I agreed with the symptoms and surrendered to them I might've become severely disabled. I truly feel that my optimism either saved my life or was saving my life on a daily basis.

We have a very difficult scenario to contend with and it doesn't offer any rational solutions.

We not only have a technological pathogen new to medicine, but we also have a technological person, new to humanity. Although we may have discovered the cause of incurable illnesses we have necessarily been forced to identify a new class of human, the artificial human.

We can count a minimum of artificial humans upon the earth by simply adding up worldwide medical statistics. And we will know that there are many undiagnosed cases as well. In addition, there will be synthetic humans whose genes have not been activated and therefore are not being targeted (on one hand this is good for the individual, but not being activated prevents an individual from reaching their true potential). In any case it would be straight forward to estimate about 210 million (3%) synthetic people on earth who have a significant illness and millions more who are otherwise healthy.

Finally, there is the question of the source of these technological pathogens. Where are they coming from? How can there be so many millions of them around the world? Based largely in my research on the androids on

Capitol Hill and my deduction that those androids were created by an advanced agency then it would only make sense that the symbions, of various classes, are being programmed by these advanced scientific races. This fits in well with my theories on manufactured realities, but not much of this will be accepted by a conventional audience. (There is also the presence of native planar symbions that are deeply rooted to the planets that are not programmed to cause disease and are dedicated to upgrading the species.)

The evidence is hard to discuss — there are quite a number of incurable diseases. These diseases have no cure and no known cause. I have presented what I think is the cause of many of these incurables. I have not done a study of each disease though have found many repeating symptoms among those diseases I have highlighted. I have added that symbions prefer technological people who have some amount of synthetic DNA. That is partly supported by three genuine and living synthetics in the American government. It seems that the only way to cure these crippling diseases is to vastly update our scientific and medicinal models. Even if we do so to be able to apply new curative techniques to previously incurable illnesses it might just be worth the effort. Instead of treating a technologically-derived symptom, we should deal with these symbion pathogens.

We should minimize these effects and to maximize the natural defences of the human body. Awareness of theses symbion attachments should prove invaluable and if we can overcome the fear and scepticism we will be able to find long-lasting cures. Symbiotes are not for everyone nor does do they answer every health issue. They may offer some relief for the millions who suffer from synthetic diseases.

MULTIDIMENSIONAL SEIZURES

There is a disorder of the brain whereby an excessive discharge of electricity changes the behaviour of the individual. The overproduction of certain neurotransmitters cause a cluster of cells to activate abnormally and the result is an epileptic seizure. About five centuries ago, the masters of the Spanish Inquisition had a different interpretation of epileptic seizures— they were associated with witchcraft and prophetic powers.

Witches practiced paganism tied to a pre-Christian era and their practices were deemed unholy. A noteworthy 1486 treatise, "The Witch Hammer" (*Malleus Maleficarum*), on witches detailed methods to take witches as prisoners and to torture them for a testimony. While the testimonies were thought to spare their lives, what happened was quite the opposite. They were punished to death.

The witch hunts, centralized in Europe, continued for about 300 years and took the lives of upwards of 100,000 witches, most of which were women. Following the burnings at the stake, epileptics were targeted again and admitted to asylums where they would once again be tortured for seizures outside of their control. Many epileptics in the United States were later sterilized in order to stop a procreative risk.

Despite advances in medicine, improved living conditions and the domestication of witches into cute and busty housewives, epilepsy has not disappeared. Perhaps 50 million people worldwide have the disorder, a disorder which has no known cause and no cure. This neurological disorder is rather unique in reality medical terms. The disorder is not inherited and yet has not disappeared in over 500 years, and it has no known cause.

This is where epilepsy, as with all our disease selections, gets interesting. Epilepsy is not just any neurological disorder. It is characterized by the smelling of burned rubber, the hearing of a buzz sound, feeling a wave of energy, a temporary state of confusion, a loss of consciousness, and possible convulsions. There may also be bits of staring, rapid breathing, unresponsiveness and eye blinks, and in some cases falling to the floor.

I've had some of these symptoms. What I also share in common with epileptics was the tingling sensation in my little finger. This tingling would spread to the forearm and then to the body. In my case there was no brain seizure and instead there was increased brain activity in the form of a download. The epileptic suffered any or all of the symptoms just mentioned.

In my personal study, I would become engulfed in a multidimensional pathogen as if a macrophage from the immune system was trying to digest cellular debris, and that debris happened to be a multi-cellular organism called a human. As I was engulfed inside of the invisible membrane, it was then my behaviours started to change, but because I could control significant aspects of my neurochemistry I would not lose control of my awareness.

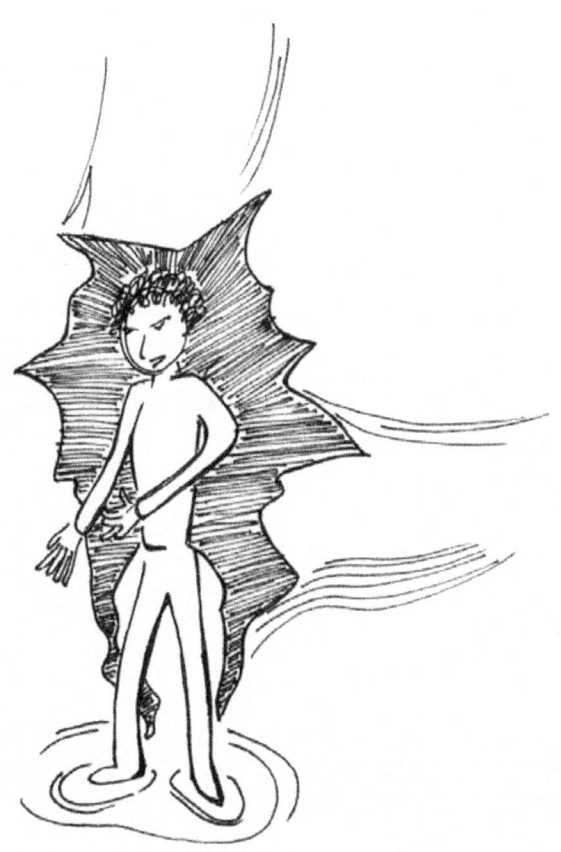

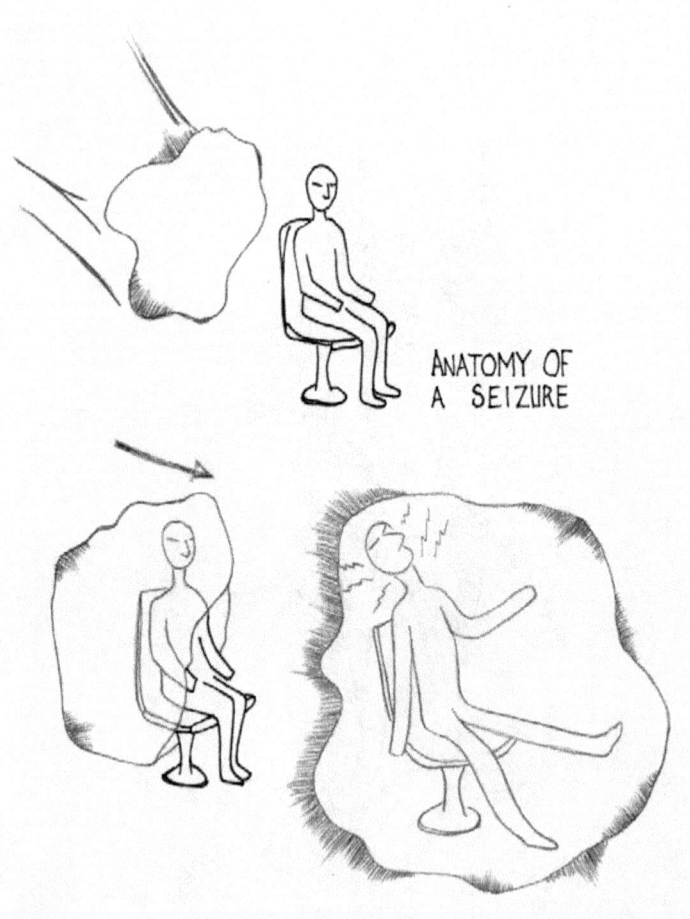

ANATOMY OF
A SEIZURE

Under some neural patterns, the symbion may teach the victim to interpret its envelope as a time for a seizure for that might easily generate a flush of neurochemicals. Oftentimes the seizure has been taught and can be untaught; that is, a person can come to the realization that the seizure is not as serious as once perceived, and sometimes even just an trained response to an illusion.

There are many kinds of seizures depending upon the size and location of this invisible pathogen. At times it can just turn into a sensory seizure — hearing the voices of people, a distorted view of reality, a spinning feeling. Even déjà vu, a temporary out of body experience, is considered a psychic seizure. In his book, *Epilepsy*, one of the world's foremost experts in seizure disorders, Dr. Orrin Devinksy, comments on the unpredictable nature of seizures. "We don't know exactly why seizure patterns change over time. There may be some changes in the brain such as reorganization of connections or an increase or decrease in the concentrations of certain chemicals."

If Devinsky's professional opinion is followed there are nearly 30 types of seizures and epileptic syndromes ranging from generalized twin hemisphere discharges to variable partial seizures. Seizures in childhood may come during bouts of high fever or the child may have a seizure followed by a viral infection and fever. In fact, fever, aches and pains, and infections will play a continuous role throughout our discussion.

You will notice almost immediately that an infection could follow or precede a brain seizure. If indeed a foreign agent is attacking the host, and if that agent is an invisible external pathogen unlike we've ever seen before, then the cause of any infection must be a result of an action taking place outside the body. In epilepsy, the side of the face that experiences numbness can change from one seizure to the next. The external pathogen can engulf the child from any direction and the direction can be detected by the tingling and numbness, or even by the drooling side of the face.

As the pathogen envelopes the child in its ectoplasmic field the body reacts and the child may experience a seizure. The seizure in this case is a reaction to survive and the electrical discharge at its root to charge the chemical constituents in the child's body so as to neutralize, even catabolises the cellular attack. This process can take a few seconds or a few minutes. A serious attack and a weak child might create a struggle of more than 30 minutes, and could even lead to scars in the brain.

Imagine for a moment a small child given a bear hug by a heavyweight wrestler. The wrestler, intent on crushing the child, applies extreme pressure to suffocate the child and the child naturally resists. In its resistance the child strains and sweats. The child is not sweating as a result from an internal disorder, as is the expert opinion on epileptics and high fevers; instead, the child is sweating and straining, even collapsing, as a result of a foreign body.

The sensations may derive from human sensory organs and neurological output, but there is a foreign organism behind the seizures. More specifically, this scenario must be reinterpreted and seen as a child being attacked by a multidimensional entity. Because the entity inhabits a higher dimension, it is unfortunately invisible to the naked eye, even invisible to the best scientific equipment. There is no known machine that can record these entities.

The administration of low to moderate doses of a drug can control partial seizures, 30% of seizures cannot be controlled, because the drugs calm the child's natural immune responses. The threat is so advanced that the human body reacts in the strongest manner possible, unless the victim has trained their immune system, and neurochemistry, as a defense mechanism.

The external agents attack only certain people, a few percent of a given population. And these ratios have remained, and possibly increased, over a number of centuries. The picture is self-determined because we have a chronic disorder that is not passed down and yet continues in the population. It fluctuates according to the size and type of organism, and according to the immunological response of the victim. It must be the case that these agents can detect certain individuals over other individuals. We know children are full of energy and their energy fluctuates by the hour as their hormones bring them closer to maturity. What if when a certain chemical fluctuation is reached the child (or adult) is targeted by one of these multidimensional agents?

A pharmaceutical drug, because it impacts a child's chemical processes, alters the child's energy signature and therefore the energy – based attack is sometimes altered. The seizure is not reduced or controlled by the drug, rather the drug affects the child's energy signature and thereby influences the foreign entity. Children of a normalized or steady signature may never attract these foreign invaders and therefore do not have epilepsy. And children who have exceptional genetics may be regularly targeted by these reality immunological responses.

Invariably some aspects of reality are releasing defense mechanisms against what it determines to be a threat or a foreign organism. That foreign organism might happen to be a child. Additionally, as a result of my work with android cultures it is also true that there are persons who can program reality and therefore they can instruct reality to, at times, attack certain energy frequencies (eg magnifying the effects of a certain virus). In doing so the people with a certain frequency or vibration may be subject to these mysterious seizures as agents are attacking them. Advanced genetics have advanced signatures that can appear on the radars of advanced agencies.

It is not an easy thing to introduce the idea that a multidimensional symbiote, a parasitic creation, could be the *cause* behind any incurable disease. It contradicts medical opinion because it clearly re-identifies the person as genetically unique (even if only temporarily) and blames a reaction or seizure on an external multidimensional (so far invisible) organism. There is proof that an external agency is present (eg the tingling sensation, numbness in cheek, fever, jerking movements) but that will not convince a medical community still rooted in three dimensional science. I can only add the fact that I have seen these energy parasites myself and have studied them with undue attention.

The only way to learn and study a multidimensional reality necessarily includes altering the frequency of energy and, as a result of my personal work with a relentless barrage of these symbiote interface attacks as well as being engulfed by these multidimensional organisms, I can attest to the fact that there is a foreign body that is the cause of many of the symptoms found with incurable diseases. Had my symptoms indeed been wholly biological I could not have recovered from any of my daily conditions. The fact that I could alleviate the symptoms by removing these parasites only reinforced the stringent principles of my reality-based healing doctrine. And all of that indeed only came about because I was not married to conventional medicine.

BRAIN WARFARE

The tingling sensation or jerky movement precedes a seizure as the viable entity slowly engulfs the subject. As the symbiotic pathogen breaks through the human immune system it hits the central nervous system. The neurological control center goes into emergency mode and responds with its neurochemical soldiers. When those are insufficient, when the brain cannot produce enough neurotransmitters to defend itself or if the person does not have adequate time to defend itself, then the technological brain drafts up additional neurological support.

The brain dials up into the reality server and downloads an app designed to counter the threat. The app is downloaded causing an electrical discharge in the brain. This releases a mass of neurochemical messages which in turn super-activates the immune system and its antibody warriors. On the surface, because the person has no training in technological human applications, there is a seizure (like trying to ride a wild horse without any horse riding lessons) from mild to severe.

A severe seizure occurs when the person does not have any capability to handle a symbiote pathogen attack. A mild seizure occurs when the person is somewhat capable, likewise, a partial seizure, even a mild one, occurs when the person is trained to process neurochemical responses, has a healthy immune system and remains calm. Whenever there is latent fear, anxiety and confusion this causes mixed neurological signals and magnifies the extent of the situation. A mild attack could end up as a severe seizure that needs hospitalization. By the same token, a severe attack from the symbiotes could be effectively controlled with proper neurological response, adequate education, and a positive outlook. The general state of health will also have a significant effect.

A healthy person is able to properly manage their internal energy, usually a healthy cardiovascular system is sufficient. When there is the onset of an attack a trained person will remain calm, activate an immunological response and moderate their thoughts (and therefore their neurotransmitters). For serious concerns a person can take an immune boosting supplement (eg high doses of Vitamin C) and increase it during certain phases of their lives.

As you can see, in a technological world there is a necessity, if not a requirement, to regulate one's state of health and not to take anything for granted. The majority of these threats will be felt by people who are genetically activated or gifted and because of their genetic disposition they have it within themselves to handle these threats. The entrance of an incurable disease can come about when a genetically advanced person avoids their innate characteristics or is uneducated in how the world really works. The world is not a biological world. The world we live in is a technological world. And anyone with advanced genetics is better identified as a technological person. The more these people maintain their body and state of mind the less likely they will ever get sick.

At times some technological people will, by accident, take a genetic leap and activate too many genes. Because they are uneducated in technological realities they will fail to adjust their thinking and will likely live a temporary high that will result in some serious disease. The disease comes about because an activated person is subject to these technological attacks and without education and awareness they will be more easily harmed.

In extreme cases, sometimes lightworkers, people who represent and spread the truth, will be the target of a malicious attack from other reality technocrats. Again, because they do not know that reality magicians are present makes them more vulnerable to harm. A reality magician, having proficiency in technological diseases, can structure a symbiote or a *symbion* to create a certain kind of disease. They can be very specific in their programming.

The same problems endure with this material because it is hard to explain to nice people that these are malevolent people who will strike them for no apparent reason. Having myself been a countless target I can assure that there are many malevolent reality magicians afoot and even you may never meet them, and may never offend them, your presence here can be offensive enough to motivate them to attack.

And if you are spreading truth and are effective in your efforts they will not hold back.

They will be happy to execute you via some surprise heart attack or brain aneurism. Failing those strange accidents they will resort to incurable diseases like diabetes or cancer. Those diseases will effectively cripple your efforts on earth and challenge your day to day living. An uneducated lightworker will be turned into a depressive, angry person who has lost their focus and their dream. An educated lightworker will not only remain positive and on the path but also an educated lightworker will use their genetic disposition to cure themselves of this technological disease long before the disease has a permanent effect.

In the calling of a technological disease there is a chance to reverse the damage and to destroy the symbion. After a certain point, the symbion will have effectively reprogrammed the person's cellular structure, weakened the mindset and instilled fear into the target. At that point there likely won't be a cure for many years to come because the program has hacked the human subject.

So this key is not only awareness and education. These are important. The next step is acceptance of the technological world. And the third step is action. An aware person needs to act in a technological manner and when they are deficient in knowledge they must seek it out and to apply it in the right way. When it comes to technological diseases there is no qualified doctor, and there is a rush to remove any damage from an attack.

The speed of the rehabilitation coupled with the proper mindset will determine the effects of an attack. The result is undeniable. If you have an incurable disease then you did not act enough. If you have avoided serious illness then you need to appreciate that you were able to prevent it and to be more careful in the future. These things can happen again as you evolve. Quite often you needn't ever be a lightworker to become a genetic target. Your presence here might cause the malevolent forces to be concerned. If you are a lightworker who has survived multiple attempts in your life the best thing you can do is to step up your mission here and to defend your body as much as possible.

Take nothing for granted and appreciate as much as you can.

The technological world is largely a thought primary world. The first comes the thought and the thought determines the genetic response. My second book *Thought Protection* discussed the importance of thought and identified early on the value of a person's state of mind. It is extremely important and is why the psychological effects preceded the physiological effects.

Before initiating a war the leaders use psychological techniques to sway the citizenry. Once they have done enough convincing then the war is possible. When too few people will agree then the leaders will use the reality system to change the root objectives and instruction of society. In both cases the thoughts precede the actions. The agreement to a military attack must precede the military attack. The smaller the attack the fewer people needed to agree; the larger the scale of a military attack the larger mindshare is requested.

It could be the case that if the immune system over-reacts that the body loses its defenses and then the symbion can invade the person. Not only is the symbion altering the molecular data and compromising the immune system, but as well the immune system is attacking itself, as is the case in autoimmune diseases.

In 1918, during the outbreak of the killer Spanish Flu, people who became infected died within hours of an attack. Experts speculated that the immune system was attacking itself as it could not distinguish between viral and healthy cells. We know that the immune system is powerful enough to combat all manner of bacterial and viral pathogens. It could be the case that the foreign agent of 1918 was improperly classified as influenza when in fact it was the synthetic symbion. Rather than a single variant, it is likely the case of a *symbion swarm* that would strike an area and infect a certain breed of humans.

We are getting the sense of a second type of symbiotic pathogen. And the symbion has another ability — it can create an immunological response. The immune system could overreact. As well, the symbion could enter the immune system disguised as a regular cell, but the cell is corrupt. The antibodies cannot distinguish between an infected cell and a regular cell and therefore attack all cells and compromise the health of the individual. There is also the prospect of multiple symbions working in tandem like a swarm of insects. The symbions could start small and then begin to expand and grow as they start to feed from their hosts.

The severe presence of symbions in your life is likely an indicator that you are a threat to the master controllers and they are dedicating their time and energy to slow down your movements or to put you in the hospital. Most incurable diseases take 10 or 15 years to manifest. During those years the symbions are wearing down the immune system and slowly deteriorating key bodily systems that will eventually cripple a human.

Not all crippling diseases strike in adulthood. Some children are born crippled and this is generally difficult to explain as well. I briefly looked at cerebral palsy in children. Cerebral palsy results from damaged motor control centers and can cause severe physical disability in children. It can occur from anywhere during pregnancy to the first 36 months of a child's life. If my theories are to hold true then we have to be able to explain how a baby's neurons can be attacked while still in the womb.

As I had done with the other disease, cerebral palsy has a number of symptoms including seizures, behavioural disorders, incontinence, spasms, and even apraxia, difficulty with facial movements (eg wink, speech). Apraxia is interesting because it involves the cerebrum, a large portion of the brain, and some classes of symbions can have a cloud-like presence that can attach itself to the human head and cause memory disturbances, speech problems, and challenges to basic tasks like putting on your shoes before your socks or putting salt in your coffee instead of sugar. Because cerebral palsy appears at such a young age (six to nine months of age) it is largely attributed to birth defects that may become evident as the baby develops. And usually there are developmental delay is these babies.

Again, a birth defect could be the result from a symbion only this parasite has gained access to the embryo. I think it totally possible to have an *intrauterine symbion* attachment. Because of this unique situation it might only have a limited functionality perhaps due to limited chemical foods and the impressive regenerative qualities of newborns. This could minimize the presence of symptoms until the child has aged 8 or 9 months.

An intrauterine attachment could also cause the baby to be born prematurely so that it doesn't die inside of the mother. A baby born into the world has a whole host of new features and defences that he doesn't have inside the womb. Up to 50% of children who develop

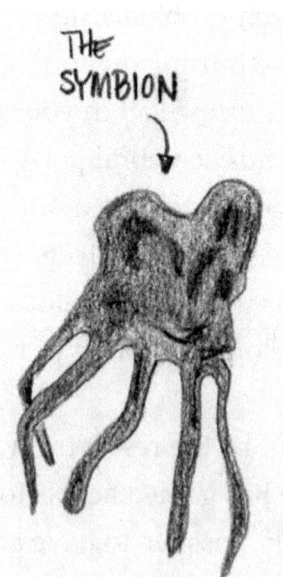

THE SYMBION

cerebral palsy were born prematurely and have damage to the brain. As we have learned, symbions like the brain and like to damage its integral functions. For reasons still unknown, a symbion will have found its way into the uterus. It might do so during copulation or it might be able to enter at times when a woman's immune system is down.

The intrauterine attachment could slowly cause deterioration and distortion to the unborn child's essential neurological processes and lead to deformities and damaged control centers. Once a person ends up in the hospital, at that point it doesn't matter — they want to cause you serious harm and it's no accident. The key is to focus on your work, protect yourself and don't let them into your mind. If they get into your mind then your health is in danger. They will try everything imaginable to get into your mind, from fear to vanity. Best thing to do is to focus on positivity and exercise moderation. They cannot harm an advanced person who lives in moderation.

They may have an out-of-body experience and feel as if they are disembodied, temporarily. Life will feel dream-like. But this may be a result of the outer-membrane of the symbion pathogen interacting with the energy fields of the human target. This is temporary because as the symbion continues to engulf the target person, the phases and sensations will shift and will be dependent upon the immune response of the person.

The brain is very sensitive to waves of energy, especially a living organism inhabiting another dimension. For example, if the outer membrane touches the temporal lobe, it could induce hallucinations, voices and as the organism touches deeper then it could include the release of memories, even strange visions. While a medical expert would say this is the result of a temporal lobe seizure and that it originates from within the deeper portions of the temporal lobe, I would not agree.

A person with repeated temporal lobe seizures would likely be prescribed antiepileptic drugs and, if ineffective, they would be recommended a temporal lobectomy surgery (removal of portions of the brain). If the symbion touches another part of the brain like the frontal lobes then the person could experience cognitive impairment or even depression. Can we afford to remove pieces of children's brains when the real cause is an external agent?

In addition to these induced seizures as a result from multidimensional symbiotic organisms, there are also going to be seizures that occur as a result of genetic deficiency or disposition. A person may have the genetic qualities that foster difficult to control seizures. As a person matures and their genes turn on and off they will experience varying degrees of responsive or unresponsive seizures.

Besides genetic disposition each person may have a physical impairment that makes them more susceptible. Some people with neurochemical imbalances will become further imbalanced as they interact with these multidimensional organisms. So there could be other rational factors that have no multidimensional component and sometimes (eg meningitis) differentiating between a physiologically-based seizure and a multidimensional one may be difficult.

Certainly, medical doctors will only have a neurological or physiological diagnosis and will unlikely support a multidimensional diagnosis until such point whereby these symbion organisms can be quantified and identified. Devinsky writes, "Anything that injures the brain or disrupts the electrical or chemical imbalance can cause epilepsy." I rest my case.

INVISIBLE INVADERS

There is a tendency with *symbions* and *symbion swarms* to internalize the effects and to get overwhelmed. It is very easy to fall victim to depression and disbelief. The human mind cannot process what it cannot understand. Certainly, the logical mind cannot accept the multidimensional organism as having any validity. The mind needs a tangible and measurable object with which to focus its attention. We are trained and educated to make decisions based on available information. In case of a symbion, the invader is invisible and this is going to challenge our perception and understanding of this material.

At the same time, having directly experienced a spectrum of these dark entities, I think that if people could see what I have seen they would never be able to sleep again. You will never see the world in the same way after you've experienced these multidimensional organisms in full color. So there is some intelligence behind their invisible quality. It took many centuries before a microscope could allow scientists to see deeper than the naked eye.

The first optical microscope was invented in the late 1500s, but living tissue was not observed up close until 50 years later. By the 1930s we had the first working electron microscope, using electrons rather than light to see an image beyond the capabilities of the naked eye. Imagine we showed people an electron microscopic view of the human skin. We would see all kinds of bacteria and cellular interactions, none of which would be pleasing to the eye. If we all had X-ray vision like Superman life would take on a whole new meaning. That is why only some of us can see environmental anomalies and these people have an obligation to share their knowledge.

If a doctor used a genomic machine to tell you exactly when you were genetically scheduled to die, it could have disastrous consequences on your life. The mysteries of life are there for a reason. Mystery and unpredictability are the cornerstones of hope, prayer, and anticipation—

all things necessary for a prosperous life. I am taking some mysteries out of life in order to drive forward human progress; for otherwise we would never be able to overcome these advanced technologies. I may only have medium intelligence, but I am gifted with a remarkable sense of wisdom.

The human brain is designed to produce chemicals in response to the observable environment and knowing everything is not the goal of life for that would make life truly boring. There are design characteristics in reality that have necessitated the need of hidden qualities. To this day, even with the commercially available microscopes, very few households actually own a microscope. That is a telling fact.

A reality is designed on many levels of interactions, what are considered to be dimensions. Not everyone has access to all dimensions. Not everyone has access to all dimensions all the time and some people have greater access. Some people get a dimensional travel card. Who gets selected isn't always easy to discern. You may truly wish to see into a higher dimension and may never get the chance.

Another person may get the chance and then wish they didn't know how life truly worked.

The difficulty with symbions is that they are working against the very people who are here on earth for a very specific reason. The people afflicted with incurable diseases are suffering from chronic mood disorders or seizures and are suffering because they have not been educated in reality medicine. They do not realize the technological aspects of reality, and they have been convinced to be afraid of out-of-body experiences.

You are not aware of these multidimensional attacks because the master controllers do not want you to know, and not knowing puts you and your child at a disadvantage. If this situation were to continue, the planet would remain the prison that it is because the genetically gifted people would be technologically compromised or crippled, and none of it is perceivable. There is very little evidence. To the trained person, the evidence is in plain sight — diseases and disorders without cure or cause. To an untrained mind, these are tragic diseases and people who get them are unlucky.

The purpose of this book is not to scare you. Some of you may become scared for a time, but I know that you will overcome it. If you can see these multidimensional entities then you can see them for a reason and your time on earth has an unearthly reason. The more you accept that the easier your life will be.

If you cannot see these pathogens there is nothing wrong with it, and, in my view, you don't need to see them to improve your situation in life. At minimum you will need to feel their presence. You will need to develop your energetic capabilities so that you can feel the presence or effect of a symbion or swarm of these reality programs. Then you can associate your senses with your observations — you can sense a dark symbion on a man's lower abdomen and then you can see that the man has prostate cancer. You can see a woman with severe depression and then also determine that she is engulfed inside the membrane of a multidimensional ectoplasmic pathogen.

People suffering from these chronic illnesses and pains now have a new cause to examine if indeed the cause of the illness is related to these multidimensional programs then there might indeed be a chance to discover a cure. Once a person experiences a paradigm shift they may discover an entirely new kind of solution.

The world we live in still cannot tolerate hallucinations and voices; people cannot understand paranormal experiences; and doctors haven't the education to prescribe for invisible agents. How you resolve your long-standing issues is up to you and as it is your life you should be open-minded to all probabilities. The kind of people who will read this book and still find it interesting after page 10 are the kinds of people who are genetically gifted (or determined to find a cure).

Normal people are less likely to read this book and having read it will easily present some harsh comments. But this is to be expected. This book is not written for normal people. It is meant to address the chronic suppression of esoteric knowledge and I am introducing some of this lost knowledge so that people will no longer remain a victim to advanced cosmic imperialists.

If any of the research from Dr. Douglas Fields, author of *The Other Brain,* is to significantly advance our understanding of the technological human then the understanding of glia, wireless cells that make up 85% of all the cells in the human brain, is paramount. Glia not only can sense electrical activity but they can also direct electrical activity in the brain. They form a powerful communication glue and have impressive regenerative qualities.

"Schwann cells (a type of glia found in the peripheral nervous system) were found to secrete a large number of protein factors at the injury site, including NGF. These neurotrophic factors are well-known powerful medicines made by the body that rescue neurons from death and stimulate and guide the growth of the severed axons," says Fields. NGF stands for nerve growth factor, an essential regenerative factor occupying the nervous system. The nervous system has an impressive ability to regenerate cellular damage. "In effect, Schwann cells sensing the injured axon reverted to an early embryonic stage to set the clock back and reinitiate the events that formed the nervous system in the first place."

If the neurons are like integrated circuits and synapses are the transistors and axons are the neural wires then glia, the largest component of the brain (and nervous system), is the wireless internet that predetermines everything. Chronic depression, schizophrenia, and mental illness have been shown to be a result of a loss of glia (oligodendrocytes and astrocytes).

There are four main types of glia: Oligodendrocytes (brain), Schwann cells (body), Astrocytes (brain), and microglia. The several types of glia serve different aspects of the nervous system and play an integral role in neurological health.

The breakdown of neurons and the demyelination (loss of essential insulation) of the axon wiring can lead to neurological disease. And the use of opiate drugs (eg heroin, morphine) activates opiate receptors in glia that release substances specifically designed to reduce the pain-relieving effects. Active astrocytes and microglia command other biological compounds such as prostaglandins to join in the fight against the opiate. The glial response to prolonged opiate use is an increase in opioid receptors in order to form a drug tolerance mechanism. They are able to adjust cellular responses in order to maintain brain equilibrium.

At birth, a child doesn't have any myelin, there's no insulation to boost the strength of their brain's signals. As the myelin grows so too do the links to motor neurons, speech abilities and then at the hippocampus — memory. It isn't surprising to know that a child has no memory before age three. If the build-up of myelin put the brain online then the demyelination takes the brain offline. Schizophrenics, on the other hand, have abnormal myelin-associated genes. The speed of the neural net is a function of its myelinated axons.

The "schizophrenic brain" could be able to alter myelin in order to create new highways of information processing depending on need. Damage to the network, for example demyelination, would interrupt the flow of information and that interruption would be experienced as thought distortions (ie hallucinations, anxieties, delusions). A symbion attachment only needs to modify the glia cells around the myelin to produce the symptoms of mental illness, and if the deterioration is significant enough this could crash the neural network, and the body.

"Glia are engaged in a global communication network that literally coordinates all types of information in the brain: glial, hormonal, immunological, vascular, and neuronal," says Fields. Glia can hear everything and then respond. Just tell the glia what to do. If the symbiote influences the glia then, for example, the glia reduces dopamine or increases dopamine. The real problem with glia suggests Fields is that "we lack the vocabulary and knowledge to speak about them in anything but general terms."

If a corporate internet is hacked, a motivated computer programmer can make significant changes to the network and even to extract all manner of private and commercial data. That loss of data can be used for any number of nefarious reason. Imagine if the glial network could also be hacked. We can see how the glia can direct electrical activity, so much so that they can reformulate the activities in the brain and to regenerate damaged cellular tissue. If there was a device that could tap into the glial protocols it could have any number of effects on the nervous system. Hacking the glia, in the right concentration, could reprogram a person.

Why is glia relevant to the technological symbion? According to my best research so far, and this is a continuing process, the symbion pathogens have a preference for the nervous system, and the nervous system is the control center of a human being. The symbion, having a multidimensional quality that can alter the electromagnetic fields of the brain, can influence glial cells. The glia can be commanded to shut down key neurological aspects, chiefly to cripple the communication networks in the brain. As the human counterpart loses connection to their brain — delusions, hallucinations, depression, paranoia, euphoria, aggression, jealousy, sadness, anxiety — the symbion gains a solid foothold in the human host. Of course, in orthodox circles this is a very speculative analysis, but in reality science it is entirely plausible.

I have seen and experienced enough symbionic attacks that I can confirm that indeed there is a new kind of parasitic life form living alongside us. These parasites not only feed off of human energy, but more so they require chemical nutrition and the human brain, especially, is a rich source of chemical nutrients. It is natural for this kind of parasitic device to be attracted to the most chemically abundant brains around and so it makes sense that people with schizophrenia, for example, would be an ideal choice.

Schizophrenia is a result from excess dopamine and dopamine is the kind of food for symbions. The loss of dopamine leads to depression. As the glia instruct the brain to replace dopamine depletion the person jumps back into a manic state. The symbion eats more dopamine and the host falls into depression, very much the characteristics of a bipolar disorder, only that my description does not blame a diseased brain. My description attributes the symptoms to a technological parasite.

The corruption of proteins inside the brain could lead to further deterioration of a person's neurological health. The demyelination of the axons weakens the flow of information and the appearance of plaques could lead to significant memory loss. The cause of Alzheimer's might be due to the long-standing occupation of a symbiotic entity slowly digesting neurotransmitters and other biological substances. The gradual degradation of the nervous system leads to the gradual onset of symptoms associated with neurodegenerative diseases.

I think that a progressive illness occurs when the host's glia have been compromised by excess symbion interference and the remaining glia activate neurotransmitter receptors in order to maximize its reduced chemical interactions. The neural chemistry in some brains is so adaptive and powerful that the brain retaliates and begins to compensate for the presence of an attached foreign body.

The symbion stimulates the neurotransmitters in the brain. The excess chemicals in the brain then antagonize and activate other chemicals. The symbion attacks are usually accompanied by fear and overwhelming negativity so they not only are carrying across a lower vibration and weakening our cosmic connection but also their tentacles are likely tapping into the brain structures such as the amygdala, a source for emotion and fear.

The target of these multidimensional organisms is only one type of person—a technological person. The more technological the person the more an attack can overwhelm. We are talking about 3% of a given population, three people in 100. Unfortunately, the effects of a symbion are disguised as psychological, neurological, medical and other speak. Carl Bazil, author of *Living Well with Epilepsy and Other Seizure Disorders* writes, "Distortions of time or space can happen: like Alice in Wonderland, the person may feel that she is becoming smaller and smaller or larger and larger."

The prevalence of epilepsy may not be the prevalence of a debilitating disorder and may just be an indication of a secretive technology that we simply do not understand. Epileptics almost never suffer from schizophrenia, a condition that we have determined to be from a loss of glia. The presence of a seizure could indicate a kind of technological download, and the subsequent activation of the glia. But if the human body is believed to be a biological device then why would the brain be equipped with an electrical charge (seizure) feature? The attribution of seizures to certain individuals, even epilepsy per se, is the result of a complete misunderstanding of human design. Hidden inside the human being is an alien machine, placed there long before incarnation, dormant now for many lost centuries.

The film *Total Recall* offers an impressive metaphorical inquiry into the true human condition. The 1990 Paul Verhoeven movie starring Arnold Schwarzenegger and Sharon Stone, was a science fiction story based on the Philip K. Dick novelette *We Can Remember it for You for Wholesale*. It earned an impressive $260 million worldwide and a 2012 sequel starring Colin Farrell was green lit.

The original story was about the ordinary Douglas Quail who decided to have some new memories implanted in order to fulfill his wish to go to Mars. When he went for a treatment they discovered that he was an undercover government agent who knew some very high level secrets. In the film, the character knows about an alien technology on Mars, a giant planetary machine that can create a breathable atmosphere if activated. The hero goes to Mars and activates the alien technology and makes the Martian surface inhabitable.

What if Mars represents the internal journey of a human being and not the external space flight? The refusal of space agencies to go to Mars in the external world represents a block in the human being to travel inside and to go to the inner Mars. Going to the inner Mars would allow a person to activate the hidden machinery inside their physical body, a machinery that only they can activate if they can overcome the psychological obstacles. By space agencies delaying the external space voyage they are metaphorically crippling human evolution. Why is that? Because we cannot see the external triggers.

The internal and external aspects complement each other. This is the basic discussion on symbions. These pathogens can affect the internal machine to produce a physiological symptom. Where we have intrinsically failed (as a species) is to identify our medical symptoms as technological imbalances. Had we been able to do that we would simply go inside and improve our machines, why we would even wake them up. I think *Total Recall* could be an unconscious display placed on screen that describes a secret to human evolution.

What is that secret? The inner machine. We suffer on earth because we are not aware of the inner machine, and those who know about it are routinely removed or sidelined. Teach people to turn on their inner machines and it fundamentally changes the operations of your body. You no longer have to suffer. You can experience a profound spiritual freedom unlike ever before. In the 1990 film, the hero's journey ends after he turns on the alien machine. Verhoeven suggests at the end of his film that the hero dies, as a result of his memory implants, by employing an abrupt "CUT TO: BLACK SCREEN." I think this is not the case in real life. My observations confirm that.

Those who accidentally access, even temporarily, their inner machine often fall victim to its fearful interpretation. That fear then shuts off essential processes in the bridge between flesh and machine and a connection to the machine devolves into an epileptic seizure, mood disorder or wild hallucination. Sometimes there is a trigger involved, sleeping pills and alcohol, but because of intoxication there is a lack of control. Once again, an immense opportunity can create a harmful result. It can be part of the addictive effect — the trigger activates the machine temporarily and then the withdrawal creates severe behavioural shifts which prompts the repeated use of the trigger: Hence, alcoholism and drug addiction, just to name a few.

STEALTH PROTEINS

How is it possible that technological agents are attacking innocent people and are behind a whole host of incurable diseases? It is only possible if our understanding of the human being is incomplete. To better understand we need to dial into the human's database of life — the DNA. Discovered in 1953, the DNA is relevant to our discussion because the symbions are able to access the DNA for the symbions and DNA share one particular trait — multidimensionality.

Symbions need to influence protein synthesis in order to inflict the internal damage they intend. They may appear as magical creatures and you may read this book as a kind of semi-supernatural discussion, but I am writing it as science, albeit reality-based. These multidimensional pathogens are not fully understood. I am still in a process of understanding how they function and without further study some of my ideas have to be inferred based on probably the most thorough understanding around.

DNA is important because proteins are needed by DNA and DNA is needed by proteins. To make the building-blocks of cells, protein, the double-stranded DNA is transcribed into a single-stranded ribonucleic acid (RNA) macromolecule. Each cell contains two copies of the human genome, the entire hereditary information of an organism. Evolutionary biologist Richard Dawkins says, "The shape and behaviour of a cell depends upon which genes inside the cell are being read and translated into their protein products." Cells are essentially miniature factories equipped with machines that can make anything from any blueprint.

The entanglement of cells with symbions initiates the transcription of a gene as a response to the foreign body. The foreign body is itself an advanced program intent on taking over a certain function of the unsuspecting host. The symbion wants to slowly kill off the host in order to extract as many intracellular chemicals as possible and to access the host it latches onto the nervous system. It immediately gets to work on the DNA. If it can hack into the genetic code, and mutate it, then it can transcribe unique RNA and use that RNA to activate some of the more than 2,000 kinds of molecular machines. These proteins will be used to produce specific chemical compounds.

As well, a mutated gene can be later copied into other cells, even all the cells, but it is only utilized in cells that are read. For example, the mutation might only be specific to brain cells. The result in those brain cells are mutated amino-acid sequences. These proteins are replicated and shared among other neighbouring cells. The internal result is an area of the brain's network that has weakened. The external result is a shift in behaviour. The invisible cause is an advanced symbionic pathogen.

In 1982, Stanley Prusiner combined the terms *protein* and *infection* and coined the term *prion*. The prion is a misfolded protein template that alters the structure of the brain. It is replicated and untreatable. These oddly shaped proteins destabilize other proteins by rubbing up against them converting the neighbour into the same malignant shape. A chain reaction ensues, body's immune system responds. Prions are interesting cases because they are protein-specific infectious agents.

Beta-amyloid, a sticky and insoluble protein fragment, is partially responsible for early-onset Alzheimer's disease. Defective tau protein deposits in neurons and even in glia can also result in Alzheimer's, a disease that has no cause and no cure. Alzheimer's disease is a degenerative form of dementia that usually results in death and misfolded proteins in the brain are the likely culprits, even if not entirely. Imagine the misfolding of a protein was inspired by a symbion's reprogramming efforts. The DNA as software could be reprogrammed, or hacked, as is the case with computer software. And specific genes could be mutated and disease-specific.

Dr. Robert Marion, author of *Genetic Rounds*, started with clinical genetics in the 1970s and truly understood the close relationship between genes and health. After stating that everything in medicine is genetic, he writes: "But the truth is actually close to this statement: virtually all chronic disorders that occur in humans — including cancer, Alzheimer disease, schizophrenia, coronary artery disease, hypertension, diabetes, alcoholism, and asthma — are conditions in which a genetic predisposition combines with environmental factors to trigger a pathological response."

He echoes some of the ideas by Kandel and the environmental effects on neural pathways. That our neuronal signalling is altered by the environment and if those circuits control our genomes then our brains are the centers for disease control, literally and figuratively. The integrity of neurological health determines just what kind of disease will manifest, from none to the deadliest kind.

With multidimensional symbiotes added to this mix, as technological pathogens, we are witnessing the evolution of artificial diseases, specifically neurodegenerative and a growing list of incurables. "A change in the base sequence may lead to a change in the amino acid sequence, altering the resulting protein, preventing it from working properly, leading to a series of symptoms and signs," says Marion. As talented geneticists might be in identifying the exact gene mutation they are powerless to remedy it.

Basically any serious disease not connected to birth defect or biological hazard that requires indefinite medication as treatment is very likely a synthetic disease. Sometimes a spontaneous genetic mutation, not genetically inherited, could also have a synthetic origin. A synthetic disease is propagated by symbion pathogens. The key identifying words are "indefinite medication."

Personally, I am not against medication and strongly feel that well-researched pharmaceuticals have their place in the world (at least for now) and are well-suited for acute health conditions. What I am against and what I am truly concerned about is the indefinite use of a drug for that indicates a chronic condition, disorder, or likely disease, and my unorthodox research tells me that these kinds of diseases are likely not biologically derived and can be artificially induced.

It is becoming increasingly easier to detect neurodegenerative diseases. Some of these we are very familiar with—dementia, Parkinson's, Alzheimer's. Molecular biologists are also getting better at isolating one or more specific genes as the probable cause. I am suggesting an even more impossible task by pointing to a technological cause.

This is not the result of rolling some dice and listening to the wind, rather I have specifically dealt with these pathogens and felt their effects. Even as I write this book I have to manage the negative influences of symbions. Without proper scientific experimentation, I have to infer how these extracellular programs are communicating with the programming inside the human body.

Venter, I think, has adequately proven that molecular biologists are well on their way to building synthetic organisms on an increasingly larger scale. And my discovery of androids on Capitol Hill, also described as synthetic humans, has convinced me that Venter's advanced DNA sequencing machines are probably 1,000 years behind whatever machine created the androids.

We all share DNA with slight changes in the genetic configuration and if DNA is software then that software can be hacked. In this case, it would have to be something made of a technology ahead of conventional science.

The symbion attachments, as they are, do not require much effort to sabotage a human body. Whether they are designed to over-stimulate the bowels (Irritable Bowel Syndrome) or if the symbions want to alter the genes so as to produce self-replicating mutant RNA, it doesn't matter. As long as we can see that there is a new kind of threat out there then everyone not aware of it is susceptible to it. I am not a geneticist, not in the traditional sense — this is a forward-thinking application of artificial biology and it may require some years to properly make sense and to add more measurement, observation, and data. The better we understand our genes, hopefully, the better able we are to self-manage our deoxyribonucleic acid-based software programs.

The symbion is an external agent. How it penetrates the immune defences of the host is very novel. It introduces itself into the body by way of stealth and unlike a biological antigen (antibody generator) the symbion is able to quickly translate some available protein into some new code. Symbions enter the body as technological proteins that will trigger the release of antibodies, but because of their adaptive qualities these cyber antigens, *cybergens*, very quickly do not look foreign. They appear to mimic their environments and share enough of the molecular structures that the antibodies may not recognize the specific determinants on cells. In adopting enough of the host's genetic code in a large enough quantity that the antibodies begin to detect that its own cells are foreign and begin to destroy its own cells and tissues.

After the symbion has entered the body it becomes a cybergen. Effectively this technological protein disguises itself using an advanced form of molecular mimicry. The antibodies cannot distinguish the non-microbial agent and healthy cells and therefore begin to destroy cells and tissue. The body attacks itself. The symbion can destroy a larger host by turning the host's own weapons in on itself in specific areas and organs.

Thyroiditis, Lupus, anaemia, colitis, celiac disease, diabetes, Crohn's disease — you may be familiar with these commonly accepted autoimmune diseases. You may have one or more of them, or know someone who does. Imagine if these kinds of diseases were caused by a symbion pathogen. The specific location of a disease would give us an indication as to the location of the symbion entity.

For example, an attack on the area of the pancreas would compromise the biological function of the pancreas and could translate insulin proteins into foreign agents that get attacked by directed antibodies. The loss of insulin as a result of autoimmune destruction of insulin-producing beta cells leads to an increase in glucose and classical diabetes symptoms. Type I diabetes is fatal without insulin treatment. It develops in healthy people and has no known cause. And diabetes has an immunological origin, a perfect candidate for symbion doctrine.

Because a technological pathogen is likely causing diabetes, or contributing to it, the person must take insulin indefinitely. This is no different than a person with schizophrenia having to take antipsychotics indefinitely. But there is hope. If the symbion could be removed soon enough, and kept off, and the health of the body was maintained, then it is quite possible to see modest to complete recovery. If the cause of diabetes was indeed attributed to a *cybergenic* invasion as a result of a symbion attachment then the removal of the symbion, the "cause," should lead to recovery.

The most powerful enemy is the unidentifiable enemy. It is the mistaken friend or the wrongly accused who may take the blame for a crime they did not commit. When a foreign molecule enters the body, as in a virus or bacteria, the immune system naturally responds with antibodies and other defensive agents (eg T cells). But that is a purely biological world and we do not live in a biological world. We live in a technological world. More importantly, we have amongst ourselves synthetic people who either are 100% synthetic or have some synthetic DNA sequences built into their genomes. We add to that technological world a new kind of synthetic threat, the *symbion*.

As a new kind of pathogen able to enter the human body as a cybergen, a synthetic foreign molecule, we are now forced to rethink the cause of some diseases. I have suggested that the presence of incurable diseases is the best place to start. An incurable disease indicates the presence of a symbion pathogen and now we can say that the symbion can enter the body disguised as a native protein, but these cybergens are not native and they are designed to cause cellular destruction. The kind of illness that manifests can inform us as to where the symbion is located. Having identified a location we can find methods to either remove the symbion, or to reduce its cytogenic effects.

These cybergens want to survive and they use molecular mimicry as a powerful survival mechanism. They can lie dormant in the body (sleeper cells) for an unknown period, but quite likely these cybergens grow just large enough to avoid immunological detection so that they can begin to sabotage many aspects of the internal systems. This is not unlike an insect infestation (eg termites) that on the surface all may appear normal when it isn't.

We know that many of the incurable diseases manifest over 10 or 20 years when it is too late to reverse the effects. As well the body will fight those foreign molecules during that period and the person may experience one or more remissions. They may even find themselves cured at one point and then an environmental trigger might relaunch the disease.

We could have within our bodies these cybergens and they may be waiting for an opportunity to strike. Quite likely, it is the case that when the immune system is compromised from some trauma or negative event (eg death, loss, divorce) then the cybergen and its symbionic companion are perfectly positioned to strike. A conventional doctor will not be able to detect a causative agent because they will not have been trained in reality-based technologies. It should be noted here, if not elsewhere as well, that the symbions discussed in this book are of a very basic nature and that there are even more complex and all-encompassing symbionic threats.

Molecular mimicry is problematic for regular people because regular people usually don't own a microscope let alone an electron microscope. In other words we are facing not only a molecular situation, something that the naked eye cannot see, but we are also facing a sentient pathogen that is able to adapt and disguise itself in order to harm the host. Symbions indeed want to harm the host. This is their purpose. As well, they want to overtake the host and to partially experience a human life or they want to create havoc in the human world.

These sentient pathogens do not arise by accident and they do not cripple lives just for fun, rather they want to disrupt the human experience and to create disharmony. The human mind, rooted in a more basic medical system, will look at them as disease agents. Patients will see their illness as a test and a challenge, but there can be no mistake on my part that symbions et al are weapons against the human species, and are very advanced. They are molecular weapons and we need to learn to defend ourselves.

If we can upgrade our medical doctrines, we can virtually sever disease at the root. The relief will not only be found in families and loves ones. It will also be found in healthcare savings and we will see the reformation of the hospital system. Understanding symbions will not end healthcare. Humans will still need bandages, surgeries, and other forms of rehabilitation. What I'm hoping for is a reduction in incurable disease statistics, a reverse course for these diseases, and an increase in the number of patient remissions, and perhaps a few miraculous cures along the way.

Ultimately, the more proficient we are with this technology the more disease we can prevent and the healthier our future. While I haven't discussed the cost of reality-based healing, what is obvious is that we do not immediately require any expensive machinery, operation, or medical test. This may change in the future as people try to profit from this fascinating doctrine, but I think it should be taught as a regular school and family curriculum for free. These are fundamental health principles that each inhabitant deserves to know and each of us personally own the advanced genetic machine (your body) within which to heal ourselves. Take advantage today of this affordable and miraculous medicine.

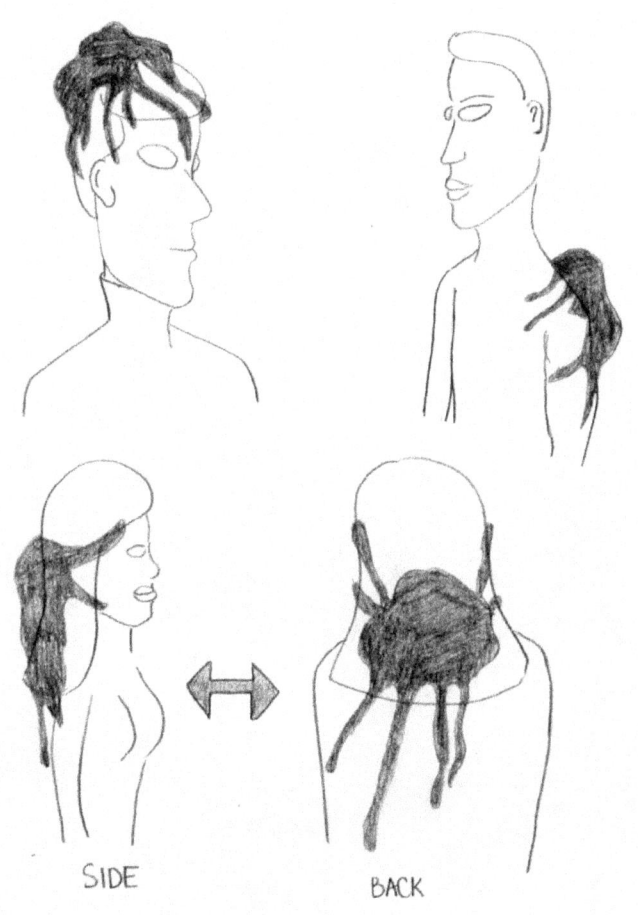

SIDE

BACK

PROGRAMMING DEVICE

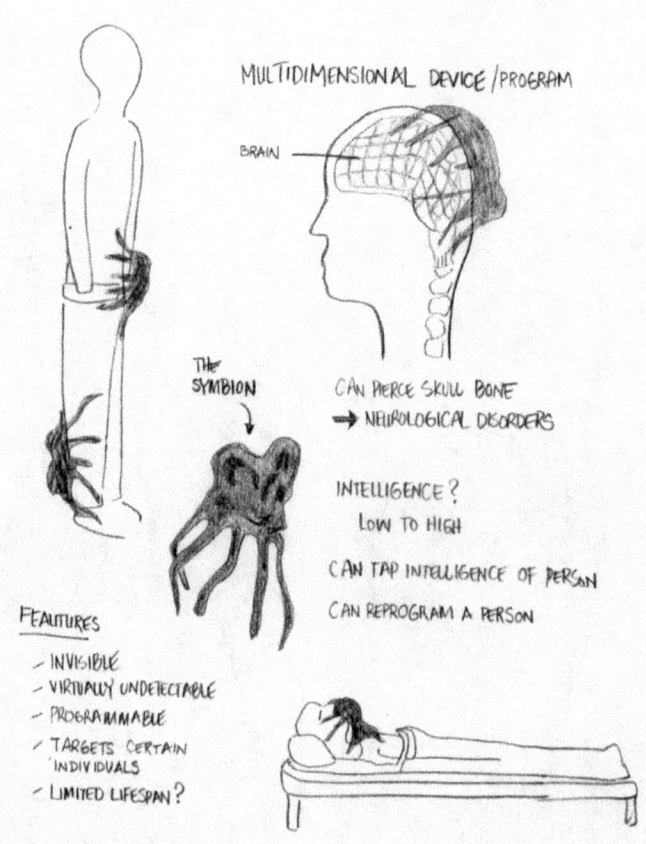

MULTIDIMENSIONAL DEVICE / PROGRAM

BRAIN

THE
SYMBION

CAN PIERCE SKULL BONE
→ NEUROLOGICAL DISORDERS

INTELLIGENCE?
   LOW TO HIGH

CAN TAP INTELLIGENCE OF PERSON

CAN REPROGRAM A PERSON

FEAUTURES

- INVISIBLE
- VIRTUALLY UNDETECTABLE
- PROGRAMMABLE
- TARGETS CERTAIN
  INDIVIDUALS
- LIMITED LIFESPAN?

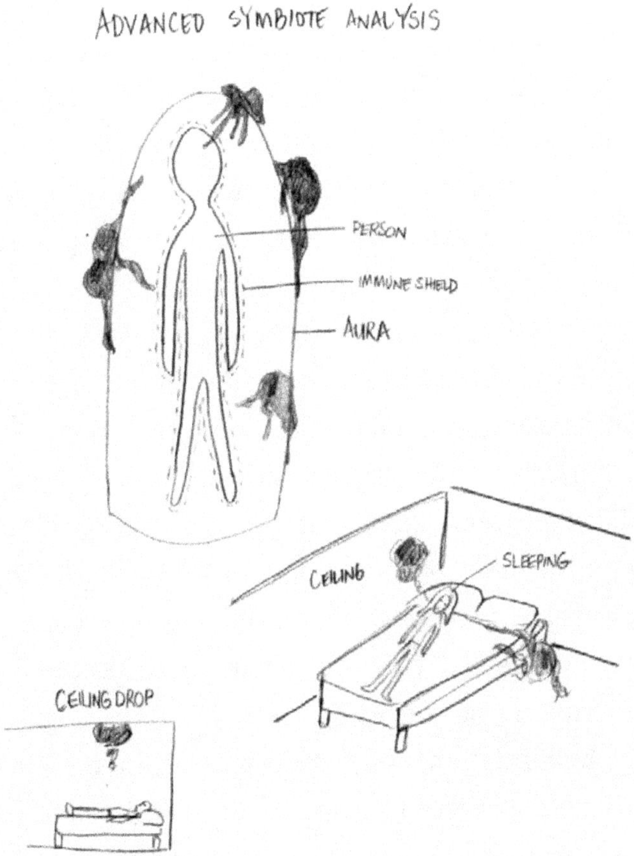

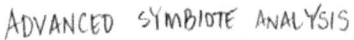

ADVANCED SYMBIOTE ANALYSIS

PERSON

IMMUNE SHIELD

AURA

CEILING

SLEEPING

CEILING DROP

INTERRUPTED PATHS

The human being can be reprogrammed to be a different gender. This can occur over the period of a childhood and it can happen over a period of weeks. The shorter the conversion period the stronger the conversion program and the weaker the immune system. The longer the period of the gender conversion, or transformation, the weaker the conversion program and the stronger the immune system. The cultural resilience of a person will have a significant impact on a person's gender identity. Some cultures are very gender specific. Some parents as well can have a very clear gender identification process.

  The kind of symbion required to convert a boy to a girl or a girl to a boy is very specific and can occur naturally or artificially. A natural conversion requires the person's explicit interest. This can be inspired by a traumatic series of life events (eg molestation) whereby the person has a disdain or distaste for who they are and then will desire to be someone else. Usually this kind of crossover takes many years. If it occurs at a young age and has support from the parents it can happen at a young age. Before there is a chance to understand the full implications of the situation the child will already have been transgendered.

A person can be convinced over many years to reconsider their gender or to dislike who they are and that will induce a gender conversion, usually at an older age when finances and independences allow it to take place. Because of the years of desire there is usually an initial relief period but later there may be issues that need to be dealt with depending on how well the conversion took place (usually there is a resistance and the presence of natural anger issues). People are in a continual state of waking and it is possible that a transgendered person may one day wake up to realize it was an impulsive mistake. Sometimes a person will fear reversion so much that they will fight waking up to their mistake. It is truly hard to predict what a person will do. The human mind is capable of anything.

I am reminded of the 1966 fictional story of Douglas Quail in *We Can Remember it for You for Wholesale*. A regular man wants a new experience and visits a company that specializes in memory implants ("extra-factual memory"). The insertion of new memories not only is designed to provide a new experience but implicit in the storyline is that the memories to be implanted will alter the person's life because it will convert them.

When Quail discovers that his ordinary life was a fake, and holding dangerous government secrets, he becomes a threat to the system. In order to prevent death he agrees to have his memories once again suppressed and replaced with a heroic fantasy set of memories. According to Philip Dick, the sci-fi author who inspired the film, it may be the case that some of his fictional works actually contained real life elements.

In a 1977 videotaped testimony held in France, the self-represented author maintains his focus as he tries to explain to the audience the revelations on the false reality he has made. He cites two books in particular: *Flow My Tears, the Policeman Said* (1974) and *The Man in the High Castle* (1962) where truth is greater than fiction. Dick references a written speech as he addresses the crowd,

"We are living in a computer-programmed reality and the only clue we have to it is when some variable is changed and some alteration in our reality occurs. We would have the overwhelming impression that we were reliving the present, déjà vu, perhaps in precisely the same way, hearing the same words, saying the same words—I submit that these impressions are valid and significant, and I will even say this: such an impression is a clue that at some past time point, a variable was changed, reprogrammed as it were and that because of this an alternative world branched off."

Dick admitted that he obtained many of his story elements from his residual memories. The science of false memories reprogramming our lives seems valid enough to write 44 novels and more than a hundred short stories. Given our new scientific thinking on memory (Kandel et al) and the presence of symbiotes inhabiting a higher dimension of reality, it is straightforward to access long-term memories and to pluck out their data. If this is true, and from my observations this indeed is the case, then it is also true that there are two lanes of data traffic and memories can be implanted. Once implanted they are likely converted into domestic proteins and the person's neurological system is quietly rewired, so much so that a person will "believe" that those memories belong to them.

What is invariably true, except for a very small number of cases (probably genetic conditions or specific birth defects), is that people do not naturally convert their gender and therefore any transgendered person is key evidence of a memory adjustment from a deep dimensional programming device, the all-new symbion. The symbion is an entirely new discovery and it is going to require some years to fully make sense of and all we have so far are these incurable diseases and extreme life choices like transgenderism.

Again, the conversion of gender cannot be achieved without a person's direct or indirect permission. If the person refuses to convert they will not convert. Of course a more potent symbion (or series of symbions apps) will likely be implemented if that is the agenda. In most of my experiences with interdimensional reprogramming, I have discovered that these entities are able to query my mind from many angles as if they compare my onboard data and try to crack my neural codes. As it makes each attempt it asks a question, each question brings it closer to cracking the code.

Naturally, I resist and I find it amazing just how persistent and it and, sadly, how easy it would be to convert people with less education on symbiotes. In other words, gaining the permission of the host isn't as difficult as it appears. The most resistant minds to gender conversion are those who were taught by parents and culture the importance of their gender at an early age. This hardwiring seems to provide some of the best defence. The most susceptible minds are those minds belonging to people from broken families or traumatic childhoods, especially where gender boundaries were crossed (eg molestation, prostitution, mentally ill parents).

There are special conversion cases in the transgendered culture. Sometimes rather than a symbion, a person will be approached by a disembodied spirit. Quite often this spirit is a reincarnated magician (or shaman and medicine man/woman), a magician who does not wish to be leave the plane and seeks out a suitable vehicle for their reincarnation. If that target is a child then it is difficult for a parent to distinguish what is really going on until probably many years later. But if the magician has reincarnated many times then they have the magical power to disguise their true identity.

The presence of a living reincarnation, the transference into a living person and not a *new* incarnation, shows some strong correlation to advanced genetic material. Only certain kinds of genomes, or genomes activated to a certain level, can process and accept a new soul, so to speak; therefore, if it indeed is a child then that child is guaranteed to have a sharper DNA base than other children and has been specifically sought out by the shaman.

The presence of multidimensional organisms does not only create a medical risk (eg depression). As well there is the possibility of being reprogrammed. It is highly likely that each person will experience at least one reprogramming in their lifetime. Some people will have many. The same deep dimensional symbions that cause the incurable diseases are used to reprogram people for any number of reasons. At times some of these are temporary, and sometimes they are permanent. In each case the permission of the person in question is necessary.

To gain permission sometimes a particular goal is promised. The promise of fame may accompany a homosexual switch. Sometimes the ending of a certain stress or pain may be offered in exchange for a switch. But because we are dealing with dark entities (synthetic parasites) aligned with dark masters, we can almost be certain that making a deal with sorcerers is a really bad idea.

167

People uneducated and unaware of these scenarios may never know what really happened and may prefer to believe that they were always meant to be the way they are (and this is intended). For example, an angelic woman is on the path to be a very powerful lightworker in the future. A sorcerer decides that a pre-emptive strike can change her path in life since one more lightworker on the path will make their diabolical plans all that much more difficult. The sorcerer offers the angelic beauty fame and inspires her to be an actor. The angelic person, usually troubled with personal issues and needing love and attention, may easily accept an easier path in life and decide to be an actor instead of a teacher. But she is choosing acting as a career because of a sorcerer's influence and also because she doesn't realize what her true destiny was.

If later she wakes up and realizes she is supposed to be a lightworker then she will be much older than expected and her positive effect on the world will have been greatly diminished. Her life as an actor will not have been in vain and may even be fruitful, but her *full* potential will not have been realized because of interference. This will usually have more serious repercussions at death when the final Life Review will come up with a poor result and the angelic woman may not have earned the right to ascend to a higher world (something she originally intended). At the human level, people don't think about the afterlife. Once the afterlife has been reached, it is too later to correct a wrong life path. In some cases a person may be freed to reincarnate and try again or may be given some spiritual tasks to make up for their failures. In any case, the afterlife is compromised.

An awake and aware person will have put aside the ego and will dedicate their time on earth to doing what they are supposed to be doing. There is nothing wrong with any profession and a person can choose any path they wish, the key is to play the right role at the right time in order to achieve the right result for the right individual. If you are being influenced and interfered with then you will have to focus to stay on the path. Almost everyone will fall off the path at one time or another, and everyone can redeem themselves when they so desire it. Denial is not a characteristic of an enlightened individual and the symbion (or sorcerer) will have every interest to maintain its own interests making these situations long and drawn out.

Human consciousness is still only poorly understood so we are not in any position to rectify everything in my discussion. I cannot provide all of the possible actions given the fact that each person is unique. The one thing that stands out is the power of forgetfulness. These advanced devices can accomplish many of their effects by employing forgetfulness. Perhaps forgetting is just the process of repressing certain genetic codes because they use it a lot and it works very effectively.

Why does it work effectively? If they want to make a little girl into a boy, in addition to implanting the boy attributes they will also make the girl forget that she is a girl. This action enhances the gender conversion (or any memory implant since it doesn't always have to be about gender). So the symbion is equipped to implant data (foreign idea) and to repress genes (forget old data). The loss of old data forces the brain to rewire itself and it bridges memory gaps by adopting the foreign idea as its own. Truly an impressive, and advanced, action.

Paris Tosen

MOOD THERMOSTATS

A release of brain chemicals causes a swing into euphoria or feelings of greatness, and worse, into bouts of anger and destruction. From a western medical perspective these episodes of mania and depression (manic-depressive disorder) belong to the newly-branded bipolar disorder. According to orthodox science, bipolar disorder is a chronic condition that is simultaneously *incurable*, our magic word and the very reason why this book has been written.

To cure an incurable disease we have to be willing to expand our thinking processes and to create a hybridized medical model. Reality medicine is my model and, as you have seen, this new kind of multidimensional medicine is short on scientific data and heavy on an imaginative interpretation of how life works. The goal is altruistic. The goal is impressive for without a new medicine these incurables are incurable.

Let's be clear, these incurable diseases are very serious. They have not only destroyed the lives of the individuals, but they have also hammered the family structure so hard that families have fallen into disarray with unanswered questions and unmanageable medical bills. Similarly, the medical systems have become overburdened and inefficient in trying to deal with incurable disease.

Drug companies are happy to treat some of the symptoms. The early antipsychotics (eg Thorazine) were not much more than tranquilizers given to people suffering from delusions, hearing voices, and psychotic episodes. But these merely replaced the electro-convulsive therapies and the lobotomies. Pharmaceuticals did not understand the mechanisms of the brain as much as they do today and were still giving neuroleptics to millions of people. Today, those powerful brain tranquilizers have become antidepressants and even administered to teenagers. Imagine the impact on a small family whose child is now taking tranquilizers and to the father who is suffering from Parkinson's and to the grandmother who has Alzheimer's. Or the single mother whose child is autistic, yet another disorder without cause or cure.

I do not take bipolar disorder lightly. I may speak about it loosely and creatively, offering the oddest sorts of perspectives but that does not diminish its seriousness and effect on people's lives. It is mostly a reflection of my own unorthodox scientific mind. Bipolar disorder, I think, has been granted the incurable status because of a myopic science and not because it is incurable.

The road to a cure is intimately intertwined in the discussion of its cause — the symbion. Bipolar disorder is a mental illness that leads to job loss, damaged relationships, an unrealistic sense of abilities, feelings of hopelessness, extreme pessimism, spending sprees, substance abuse, and hospitalization. There can be years without symptoms, flare ups, and numerous remissions. Each person might have a trigger, something that brings on the disease to its fullest effects. And up to 50% of people attempt suicide. All of this is pretty significant.

A person with bipolar disorder is a person tortured by their own thoughts. They see the outcome of life in the worst possible way when they are depressed and when in mania they see themselves as movie stars and saviours. With all that dopamine rushing through their brains they might act upon their delusions, they might all of sudden take a trip overseas just because they deserved it. Or, in the case of destructive behaviour, they might take a sledgehammer to the house of their ex-wife. And all the meanwhile the little cause, the little control device, is hiding in another dimension as it remains neatly attached to their nervous system. In my view, the bipolar person is not under self-control; rather they have been hijacked by an impressive little creature straight out of a twilight zone.

Reality science is a profoundly different application and a multidimensional interpretation. The psychotic drive into depression and pessimism is not originating from within the person rather the external symbion agent has hacked into the nervous system and is feeding off of the raw neurochemicals such as dopamine, serotonin, and acetylcholine. The drop in dopamine and serotonin then cause the mental state of the individual to drastically drop. If the symbion remains attached, the person will experience long term depression, but some people have automated defense mechanisms and will multiply the production of the depleted neurochemicals to compensate for the heavy chemical leeching.

Unfortunately, not all brains are made equal, and some people may be so compromised that they may experience a delay before their systems attempt to retake control. Awareness of the situation will immediately help the response time because the person is conscious of a neural hijacking and could wilfully control the release of a new bunch of neurotransmitters. But neurological control is a very fine art that no one is immediately expert at; therefore, the expected mood swings are present. A low is replaced with a high.

The flood of chemicals are digested by the symbion and the person, days later, returns to a low, perhaps even lower than before. A number of days later the person may attempt another neurochemical remediation. If the symbions remain, because sometimes they may appear in numbers, the individual may experience a period of challenge and if severe enough will likely turn to antipsychotic drugs, or even opiates. Illegal drugs might alleviate some of the symptoms and may lead to addiction while the symbion is never addressed.

Becoming aware of these multidimensional parasites allows people to delay the pharmaceutical remedy and to pursue a new kind of treatment. If you are a sufferer and you have determined that you are a target then it is highly likely that you have the genetics, or ability, to handle these neurological invaders. Only you will know this and since it is likely that you haven't any skill in managing your energy systems, and you didn't study neurology in school, whatever you do will not work instantly. You will need time, and years, to develop your skills in fighting symbion attacks.

Teenagers are particularly susceptible because they do not know themselves and are experiencing all manner of personal crises on a daily basis. There are countless problems with boyfriends and girlfriends; there are misunderstandings between parents; there are psychological problems pertaining to beauty and failure; and there are challenges at maintaining school grades. Teens suffering from depression are probably more common than we think. Of course, teen depression is temporary, but it can also be revolving and very polarized.

In extreme cases, depression could lead to suicidal thoughts, the feeling that there is no solution and that life is over. As serious as it is, teens should be reminded that their whole life is ahead of them and all things work out for the better. Now when symbions are present, a teenager needs to realize that they are being influenced to be depressed and there may be subtle voices who are telling them to kill themselves; therefore they should not listen to these dark voices.

Any negative inner voice that you hear is not your voice, it is the voice from some other entity, spirit, or even sorcerer. These kinds of demented, distorted, and childish creatures wish you dead because they fear your light. The dark entities do not wish for beings of light to live. No matter how bad it looks, and sounds in your head, best thing to do is to realize that there is a dark entity (bad demon) attacking you and to resist no matter what.

You can tune out the negative voices, burn a candle and some incense, do some prayer and meditation, and put on some good music. And make it a habit. Keep it a secret if you like. You incarnated here for a good reason, you made the effort, it was a lot of work, and you have to stay. No one goes home early.

People who know that they have bipolar disorder know only because a licensed psychiatrist, or similar, has confirmed it with a specific clinical diagnosis. You may have these manic-depressive symptoms but not the professional diagnosis. My position is that these symptoms can be caused by symbion attachments and by paying attention closely these symptoms can be minimized without drugs. That by strengthening the immune system and the general health of the body, and by improving the lifestyle and staying away from negative influences, these symbions may lose their incentives.

It is also true that some people are so sensitive to the environment, and their neurochemical balance is unsteady to start with, that a symbion attack isn't necessary to create any mood swings. Not every case is a result of these energy parasites and sometimes too much stress and not enough sleep is likely the cause. Some brains are born defective as well. The better you understand your body the more likely you will see what is going on. As well, the better you maintain your health the less susceptible you will be to any multidimensional attack.

One of the fundamental characteristics of an advanced species is their natural ability to appreciate spiritual growth; and a primitive species fears spiritual growth. Spiritual growth includes genetic growth; that is, the unlocking of certain genetic codes must be present in order for a person to evolve. The more a person adheres to this philosophical approach to life the less intrusive these interferences will be because the more resilient you are genetically the more stable and secure your existence.

Synthetic medicine differs wildly from biological medicine in that it understands and truly appreciates the genetic evolution of a person, and even of a culture. This is what cultural traditions are for—cultural tradition was designed to ensure culture evolution. Modern culture has been woefully corrupted by capitalism, militarism, egotism, and religiosity. There is no direct dedication to genetic evolution and in its place people just work to hopefully retire with a good pension and a big house. A person using reality science techniques is intimately aware of their genetic basis.

PARASITIC AGENDA

The symbion device appears to be one of the major causes of a wide-ranging set of diseases, illnesses, and health conditions. The symbions may be specifically created to attach themselves to certain body frequencies and given the synthetic nature of the world is probably the case that synthetic DNA is one of the key identifiers for these multidimensional parasites. It's like a heat-seeking missile that does not register objects radiating cold and is designed to target objects radiating heat.

The medical diagnosis is the greatest challenge and I think it is because of our medical education. In the orthodox medical system, probably the one in most use worldwide, each disease requires a specialist. A mental illness is given to a psychiatrist and sexual disorder is handed to a gynaecologist. But when we are dealing with symbions — invisible parasitic organisms with ectoplasmic qualities — we have to step outside of orthodoxy. Why? Because a symbion attached to a person can create multiple symptoms to deal with; therefore, multiple specialists will not be able to make the connection unless they all sit in the same room to discuss the patient's total number of illnesses.

With a single symbion attached to the back of the head and with its tendrils deep into the brain stem or basal ganglia, central aspects of the nervous system, could very easily produce depression, arthritis, and fever all at once. A larger symbion could deplete the dopamine reservoirs enough, given time, so as to artificially induce Parkinson's or even Alzheimer's. And if it remains attached the patient will never be cured and will be on medication indefinitely. People with schizophrenia must take antipsychotics indefinitely. People with diabetes have no cure. Without revising the medical system we will only see the proliferation of these mysterious and incurable illnesses and the continuation of pharmaceutical drugs that are not resolving the source of the illness—multidimensional parasites.

The arguments against my arguments are valid. As much as my illustrations and discussions may prove to be illuminating the case remains that the cause remains invisible except to probably a handful of people. I have seen the symbions and all the other paranormal entities I have spoken of. I am aware of a select few who have seen similar things but did not understand what they had seen.

I also understand that these creatures are pretty frightening and they enjoy debilitating human memory systems. They can easily tap into the hippocampus' memory banks and alter memory so that people who witness them want to forget what they have seen. The auric fields that they can effect also have an impact on the emotional sensors found in the amygdala and the target will be afraid to even consider the idea that an invisible parasite has invaded their multidimensional body.

This book is still a preliminary discussion, but according to my observations and experience so far I would have to say that, aside from defects and injuries, human disease has been artificially induced using a very advanced technological application. Sadly, there are agencies inhabiting deeper dimensions that are behind the administration of disease and because society is wholly unaware of how reality works it is also true that disease will remain indefinitely.

What is also clear and something that needs to be pointed out is one important fact—if diseases can be artificially induced, even incurable illnesses, then it is also the case that all diseases can be cured. The cure for all disease lies in understanding how symbions interfere with the systems of the human body because that will teach us how to manipulate our bodies, our very DNA, so as to combat the parasitic effects of these genomic hijackers. In addition to that seemingly impossible task, by improving our innate genetic disposition we just might be able to peer deeper into reality and could more easily spot these hidden scientists and controllers.

I do not casually say that I think I have found a cure for these striking diseases. What is certain from more than six years of firsthand experience with multidimensional parasites (symbions) is that human disease, probably all or most of it, is being induced by an advanced technological application. More than ever we need to pry ourselves away from clinical diagnoses and drug therapy and to study the concepts I have presented in this book.

I do not think we should cut out drugs. I think that we should add to the diagnosis the possibility that a technological parasite, of ranging qualities, classes, and complexities, is behind a complex and mysterious disease. I am confident to say that, in particular, incurable diseases would benefit from my research, and since these diseases have no cure then a new approach may indeed be welcome.

Why would some advanced scientific cultures be spreading disease among the human population? That is a most difficult question to answer and it fundamentally sits behind my extensive work in android theory. Again, as I have stated, we live in a technological reality and therefore all things are in fact technological, including the human body. The better we understand that the faster we can eradicate disease. Imagine how much better the world will be without cancer, without dementia, without mental illness and without the seasonal flu.

I did not foresee myself reaching a point of observation that would include the statement, "All disease is artificially induced and I think I have found the cure," and, at the same time I have directly interacted with symbions for a number of very difficult years, and still do today. I do not speak lightly of disease nor do I suggest that it is easy to combat symbion technology. My focus is on specifics: there is a technological cause for disease and incurables, especially, as a result of symbion attacks.

Removing the symbions and modifying the genetic circuitry should lead to, at the very least, an improved state of health, and quite likely, if the damage isn't permanent, to a remission and a permanent cure. We are no longer battling viruses and bacteria agents; we are now battling multidimensional symbions that use our own cells to produce virus-like cells. (I am not omitting real live viruses that we pick up from the external environment.)

Symbion, an advanced multidimensional pathogen that can reprogram the nervous system and artificially induce disease in its unsuspecting host.

Welcome to the next era in human medicine. If there was a time for human medicine to make a leap forward, this is the time. By reducing disease we necessarily reduce the burden on natural healthcare systems, we ease the work of doctors and alleviate health insurance premiums, and we just might make hospitals profitable.

This multidimensional pathogen is able to overcome many of the immune system's primary defenses and to attach itself to key areas of the central nervous system and thereby begins to cripple the normal human processes. The parasitic prowlers feed on dopamine, serotonin, acetylcholine, and other essential chemicals like calcium, glutamate, and magnesium. As the human host is slowly taken over they begin to become ill and soon develop one or more incurable diseases.

These ectoplasmic agents feed off of a human host, even to tap into the human intelligence so as to take over the person. A person who has been properly hijacked will find themselves deep into some kind of inescapable addiction, criminal behaviour, or violent tendencies. Some of these multidimensional agents can convert the sexual identity of the host and make a straight person gay and a gay person bisexual. It is very likely that people suffering from sex addiction, and even strange sexual practices, are doing so as a result of an attached symbion agent.

Symbions are not cellular organisms like viruses and they do not have the DNA of bacteria. At this early phase of discovery, the symbion pathogen appears to be composed of ectoplasm, a higher dimensional reality substance, or a divergent form of arvicity. The symbion can manifest into a synthetic DNA-based organism, enough so, that can make contact with the human spiritual body.

In other words, the human spirit's composition can be matched, to some degree, by these multidimensional agents. This allows them to supersede the physiological defence mechanism, including the immune system. Once the symbion enters the human host it extends a range of tentacle-like arms and hooks into the control center of the human machine: the central and peripheral nervous systems.

The human body is extremely resilient and has many unknown defense mechanisms. It isn't easy for the symbion to accomplish its tasks, but considering the virtual lack of awareness it is only a matter of days or weeks before this technological pathogen has gained a foothold. It stays alive by feeding off of chemicals with the body, especially neurochemicals (and their energy output). Some symbions may feed on the circulatory system by hacking into the spleen and liver pathways and causing the host to be artificially anaemic as molecular energy in the blood cells are depleted.

The symbion is an entirely new interpretation of some ancient evil entities. It is very likely that these evil pathogens have been around for thousands of years and somehow have been tolerated. This has not always produced a positive result. People who were driven mad, for example, may have been crucified in early times, and, later, they may have been improperly placed in an asylum. Symbions attached to the frontal lobe of a target may have led doctors to lobotomize the host without realizing that the person had a unique pathogen attached to their etheric body. Some women may have been burned at the stake because the Church felt she was possessed by the devil when in fact she may have been overcome by a powerful program.

The true strength of the symbion is to conquer the host from the inside out, sort of like rust. The rusting of a metal is an electrochemical process whereby a chemical agent corrodes (or consumes) the exposed metal until there is either no more oxidants or no more metal food. The symbion begins to convert the cellular composition and protein structures in the host's body chemistry so that the host's own cellular data begins to attack itself. Because the host is now attacking itself the immune system cannot distinguish between the causative agents and the damaged cells. The condition for an autoimmune condition are perfect. For example, antibodies mistake the body's own cell proteins for an invading bacteria.

What probably occurs is that the symbion corrupts a protein and converts it into a foreign molecule. Rather than a virus or bacterial cells, the body is spontaneously invaded. The antigen (cybergen) grows and triggers the production of an antibody. But the irregular antigen shares many characteristics of a regular protein; and therefore can negotiate (or fool) a longer residency. (An epitope, foreign molecule, and a bacteria appear so similar that the antibody — B cells, T cells — cannot tell them apart. The result is that the immune system begins to attack the body.)

Once a symbion has "negotiated" a stay on the host it can then feed off key chemical nutrients and to slowly take over the target, depending on the programming of the pathogen. Each symbion has a different cellular program and quite often there are multiple symbions on a host. Sometimes the symbions can merge together and synergistically multiply into a larger symbion that is more akin to a dark entity than a simple multidimensional pathogen. Usually we can infer the kind of symbion attachment based on the degradation qualities of the host.

There are likely a number of key classes of symbions that can be identified at a later date. The word "symbion" is derived from "symbiote," an organism involved in a symbiotic relationship. The symbion cannot live very long in the dense reality by itself, or, it must exist in a more innocuous format. As it finds a host it is able to feed and grow then to slowly corrupt the host as it is programmed to do. It is a kind of *ectosymbiosis*, only that the body surface is the spiritual (etheric energy) body.

People with Tourette's syndrome, considered an organic disorder, have to manage unexpected tics and vocalizations. Drugs are used to suppress the neurotransmitter dopamine and this is believe to reduce some of the uncontrollable movements. Strangely enough some of Tourette's sufferers can modify their symptoms and even to suppress their tics and unintentional vocalizations. Dr. Oliver Sack, author of *The Man Who Mistook His Wife for a Hat*, describes a case where a man with Tourette's symptoms makes his symptoms disappear when flying a plane.

In my unscientific approach, a person's bodily frequency must necessarily shift into a higher mode as they engage in some important activity. When the activity is done the frequency drops down to a steady state. If Tourette's is anything to go by then we could say that the symptoms are bothersome in a low frequency and can be overcome in a higher frequency.

The attachment of a symbion on the basal ganglia, the area responsible for some bodily movements, functions only at certain frequency of vibration; therefore, as an afflicted person focuses and engages into some important activity the symptoms seem to vanish. In fact, the symptom of Tourette's syndrome do often wax and wane for unknown reason. At times, they can even disappear. From a reality perspective, much of this has a lot to do with a frequency shift in the person. A higher frequency minimizes, even alleviates the symptoms. This can occupy minutes or hours at a time. Similarly, the objective of the symbion is to remain in control and it only can remain in control at a lower frequency of vibration and it will make attempts to undermine the frequency of the host because at a lower frequency it has greater effect.

A disease, any disease, can be progressively worse and that means that deeper aspects of the human physiology can become permanently damaged. The early presence of a symbion is the best time to remove and nullify its effects because as it engages the architecture of the host it begins to reprogram the host and that is when certain systems, and organs, are compromised. A person who has lived for many years with a number of parasitic attachments has very likely lost some of their regenerative capabilities. For example, a Parkinson's patient of 20 years may have a damaged substantia nigra and even if the pathogens are removed, if indeed they are there, he may not be able to return to normal.

Clearly, the Tourette's sufferer has very likely been taken over by a symbiotic agent, or multiple agents. The agents are intelligent and they can access the host's thought channels; therefore they are prone to communicate to the host. Symbions, in general, are negatively charged (or evil) and are designed this way in order to corrupt (or hijack) the good-natured human. A good human is a perfect target for a negative entity.

The symbion jams the host's thought channels and signals as a process to compromise the host. They can also lock the thought channels to specific energy quotients (genetic combinations). That means that whatever memories are associated with those quotients will be broadcast.

In some ways it is like the dial on the early television set with a 500-channel network. Along those 500-channels, many of the programs are pretty boring, violent, or repetitive. Imagine every so often your service provider locks your television programming on adult entertainment, and you are helpless to change the channel. What you are forced to watch — because you have to watch TV — are nude people performing restricted acts. Imagine still that you had kids at home, and the TV was on because it can't be turned off, and they had to see naked people acting badly.

People with Tourette's are prone to blaring out coarse and foul language. This is either streaming directly from the foreign entity or it is from the locked channel. The natural communication channels can block or tune out the foreign signals, most of the time. The presence of tics and other unintentional movements are a result of the symbion's connection to the basal ganglia. As its presence becomes more secure the Tourette's symptoms might get more intense.

While fear of public humiliation may be prevalent and of concern to a person, invariably the road to a cure requires a fearless attribute because a fearless attitude disagrees with the symbion's programming. The symbion instils fear, doubt, and confusion into the host in order to weaken the host, because a psychologically weakened host is easier to take over. A person with Tourette's, and any serious disease, can defeat the symbion pathogen(s) by adopting a positive attitude and by maintaining a higher frequency of existence.

If the person is afraid of being in public then it is imperative that the person goes out in public. People who confine themselves to their home, or room, will only increasingly become a slave to the foreign entity, and may end up being hospitalized. If the host (the person) refuses to face their health challenges they will likely be completely taken over at which point they will expire. The symbion will leave the host and find another.

REPRESSED PREDISPOSITIONS

When the symbion interfaces with the host it has no predetermined result. The outcome of these multidimensional pathogens attaching themselves to the etheric body (spirit body of a human being) is determined after a negotiated attachment. It is largely decided by the native disposition and demeanour of the person. For example, a woman with the occasional hysteria may become a subject to fits of hysteria that are so extreme that they could include suicidal tendencies. She may try to poison herself under an attack. On the other hand, a woman with occasional melancholy may be subject to fits of heavy depression which may require medication.

The symbion pathogen, in many ways, is limited by the composite of the human consciousness. In special cases though, and with certain types of people, the symbion could completely override the human interface and literary hijack the body. The symbion could drive the body into drug addiction and can also turn the person into a violent killer. Some murderers, obviously not all cases, commit murder (or even rape) in order to satisfy the incessant command of the symbiotic entity.

The entity, driven by base malevolent desire, will take advantage of the divine spirit and will enjoy raping a child or murdering someone. Later, the person will not be able to rationalize what happened. The closer in line between symbion and host the more likely this process will be continued. A psychotic individual fixed with a malevolent entity may enjoy each other's company, and will deny, lie, and deceive in order not to be caught.

The symbion—entity, parasite, pathogen, program, device—magnifies and distorts that which already exists inside of the person. It also tries to sharpen certain critical negative aspects to make them more severe and more refined. A person with violent tendencies could become a mixed martial artist with episodes of going berserk. The host will then likely study fighting arts, perhaps even competing, as a means of satisfying the needs of the entity. It is a very fuzzy and often confusing line that could take many years to understand — who is controlling who? Is the symbion (entity) controlling the host (human)? Or is the human in control and his lifestyle is just a result of his native disposition?

Oftentimes we cannot know and the only person who really knows is the afflicted individual. Given the survival needs of the entity, it will tell the human mind to lie and deny as much as possible. Quite likely the host will never know unless they have adopted an ascetic lifestyle free of most of life's attachments. Only then can they explore who they truly are.

The symbion is intelligent to some degree and is also programmed for specific tasks like violence or paranoia. When they tap into the human neuron system their intelligence gets a boost as they borrow from the larger microprocessor. Slowly they learn the disposition of the host and conceive a way to negotiate control.

The symbion has a child-like mentality. It is strictly an egotistical being with a limited existence (it needs a multi-cellular carbon-based host). It doesn't care what happens to the host's body. If it latches onto a woman and inspires her to become a prostitute who then gets addicted to heroin (or methadone), that is fine. Remember, the symbion only cares for its own survival.

It is like a carjacker. The thief steals someone's valuable car and goes for a joyride. The thief has no concern what happens to the vehicle. If this one breaks they can hijack another one. Only in our case we are dealing with human lives and families who love one another. We are also dealing with an invisible thief that is more prevalent then we have ever known. In some ways this is a kind of possession, and in many ways it isn't. Why? Because the host and the symbion have negotiated an agreement (even if the host is unaware of it, as is usual).

When a more powerful symbion is present, it can actually augment the host's psychic abilities, even to give it the power of prophecy and intuition (along with delusion and disinformation). This may be done in order to make the host compliant. "If you let me stay, I'll give you superpowers." For difficult subjects a stronger symbion may be used to win them over. They could make them a better actor, causing them to win audiences, or, they could make them a stronger fighter, causing them to gain more respect in the street.

These negotiations are often very subtle; small voices in the middle of the night; a choice in the middle of a dream; or even an opportunity for success. Each person has wants and desires that the symbion can access. Sometimes they can search the memory banks in the hippocampus and determine an effective negotiation strategy. As long as people remain unaware that an invisible thief may be attached to their nervous system they'll often end up playing the victim and may lead a misguided or small life.

Symbions, simple-minded creatures who enjoy pleasure, have a vampiric nature and need to feed. Their favourite foods are found inside the human body, chiefly in the brain. They feast on neurochemicals in particular, among other chemical nutrients. They usually drive the host into situations that will release more neurochemicals and hormones. One simple way to create an instantaneous buffet for themselves is to entice the host to have an orgasm. The orgasm is guaranteed to release a mass of fresh neural juices. Problems with excessive masturbation could be attributed to an attached symbion. People who prefer sex over masturbation will likely find themselves involved in casual sex situations. More often than they should. Not all cases are serious. Quite often a person may even enjoy living a more adventurous life or may like masturbation. The symbion could be a sexy person's base needs as well.

Host and symbion together create new forms of psychopathological behaviours. Clinical observation and study of these behaviours likely contribute to additional psychiatric illnesses and conditions. On the personal level though life could very well become bipolar and the original identity of a person may get lost for periods of time. These behaviours may be explained as co-dependency, psychosis, repressed emotions or even degenerative inheritance.

In early cases of Tourette's in France, around the time of the twentieth century, Meige and Feindel developed a guide "for the treatment for persistent tic and obsessive-compulsive behaviours that addressed both the variety of symptoms and the differing course and outcomes experienced by those displaying these symptoms," writes Kushner in *A Cursing Brain*. Kushner goes on to describe an idealised patient sample, or, who was a tic patient with both an "extraordinary intelligence" and "infantile regression."

Meige and Feindel believed that the cause of tics was a result of a person's infantile behaviour. Yet, at the same time, they acknowledged that a person with tics (or Tourette's in modern times) had extraordinary intelligence. One of the key methods of subversion from the symbion is to use the host's own molecular infrastructure against them. They turn a protein into an anti-protein that still looks like the other proteins. Symbions use mimicry to survive and thrive, as do children, what Meige and Feindel describe as a "lack of will." It is ironic that in 1902, in the very early phases of discovering Tourette's, doctors were commenting on the infantile nature and restlessness of grown men with tics.

These early physicians did not realize that infantile symbions could have caused the wild gesticulations of a man with tics. The patient may have had a symbion that initiated him so much that is caused his unruly behaviour. Because tics patients are also described as being able to focus and remain calm during events they enjoy like fishing and billiards.

Freud himself studied convulsive tics in the late 1800s. Her name was Frau Emmy von N., a forty-year old woman with hallucinations and convulsive tics. Freud determined that the woman suffered from hysteria, overwhelming emotion (usually fear), as a result of repressed childhood trauma. Imagine that the woman's nervous system had been compromised by a parasite. The entity, with tentacles extended well into the key brain structures, has a tangle in the memory device, the hippocampus.

The woman, completely unaware, would have spontaneous recall of her childhood traumas which would cause her to contort her face in horror and to make some ungodly sound. Freud's psychoanalytical approach would notice the activation of repressed memories but would not notice the presence of a multidimensional symbion. He would teach her to come to terms with her repressed traumas and the woman's condition would improve. What hasn't been dealt with is the cause of the resurfaced memories — symbions. The woman would have relapses and a continued state of generalized phobias, likely attributed to a technological pathogen well outside of even Freud's perception.

As we are seeing, the mental predisposition of the person is an elemental determinant upon the causative result from a symbiotic attachment. And since each individual is uniquely predisposed with their own set of traumas and hidden desires, we get a wide variety of mixed symptoms and medical arguments between physicians. Is it a mental condition or a separate disorder? Was the behaviour an uttered expression of some repressed desire or just childish impulse?

Tics too seemed to follow a similar symbionic pattern because they developed after an infection. As we discussed earlier, after the symbion finds a host and invades, their first task is to corrupt some molecular data, causing an infection, and then to negotiate an agreement. Following that process we see the evolution of various symptoms like tics and hysteria.

Case in point: the global epidemic of encephalitis lethargica (1916-1930) not only put many people to a lengthy sleep but those that remained awake developed tics. The movie *Awakenings* starring Robert DeNiro and Robin Williams, and based on the memoir of Dr. Oliver Sacks took place in a hospital of comatose patients in 1969, all of whom were struck with encephalitis lethargica in the 1920s. Under Dr. Sack's experimental care, he managed to wake a male patient using the Parkinson's drug L-dopa (synthetic dopamine).

As the patients were administered L-dopa they would awaken and many would have wild, uncontrollable tics and jerking movements. Encephalitis lethargica was also an infectious disease of particular importance to my discovery of android cultures on Capitol Hill since the disease had no cause and no cure. This mysterious sleeping sickness struck a large population for about 15 years and has never since returned. And it depleted the neurotransmitter dopamine, chiefly inside the mid-brain structure known as the substantia nigra.

The substantia nigra became a shared brain structure also found in my living androids. In other words, both the android politicians and the comatose encephalitis victims heavily relied upon the nigra structure. I concluded that since the activated nigra, rich in dopaminergic neurons, in the androids gave the androids life then it was likely the case that the depleted and damaged nigras in the encephalitis patients proved that they too must have been androids.

Looking at Tourette's syndrome I cannot help but see an abundance of shared similarities common to my android research. The ticcing and vocalizations of the Tourette's patient not only tells me that they are attached with some symbion species, as well, and probably more importantly so, people with Tourette's are likely as well androids. This would explain their shared similarities with encephalitis survivors, and even with people with Parkinson's, and the survivors of encephalitis share the substantia nigra with the android politicians.

The mysteries of incurable diseases are becoming less and less mysterious. Fundamental to the conversation are some pretty inventive elements — symbions and androids. By the same token no medical professional or machinery has been able to solve the mysteries of a handful of incurable diseases. It would seem that the cure rests in a reinterpretation of not only the nature of reality but also of the disease. Rather than trying to cure an incurable biological disease; instead, we are to position ourselves to cure an artificial disease.

The biological disease has no cure because it is nonbiological. An automobile cannot be tuned up using antipsychotic medication; rather an automobile requires a qualified mechanic with a specific set of tools. We have found no cures for some diseases because we are using the wrong set of tools and that is because we wrongfully believe that we are facing biological illness when in fact we are not. The medical field employs both biological (body) and psychogenic (mind)

explanations of a syndrome. I am now offering a
third approach: technological (DNA)
explanation.

CASCADING DEGRADATION

If we use a clinical approach to the presence of psychosis (hallucination, paranoia) in a person with an incurable disease we are forced to explain these disturbing behaviours using logic and rationality. We apply our social skills to try to calm down the psychotic turn of events. Failing the nondrug approach we inevitably find a new drug prescription for the patient. Alzheimer's patients, for example, have to deal with psychosis in addition to lapses in memory. Nearly half of Alzheimer's patients have psychosis. Western medicine cannot completely answer why people with Alzheimer's easily become irritable, cannot sleep at night, suffer from anxiety and depression, except to say that the general decline of the brain is cause for more complications. The cause of depression in Alzheimer's is Alzheimer's, as is the cause of insomnia and psychosis.

Forty percent of people with Alzheimer's experience a distorted sense of reality such as seeing people who aren't there and having paranoid suspicions that lack evidence. A build-up of beta-amyloid plaques begin to clog the neural wiring. Short-term memory begins to lapse increasing to longer-term memory. The person begins to become more uncertain and foggy and the incurable disease becomes irreversible. The handful of drugs that can slow down the symptoms are often administered too late. Researchers in Rotterdam have recently discovered an elevated protein in women that could alert them as to who would be more likely to develop Alzheimer's.

The application of symbiotes to neuro-degenerative disorders presents an entirely different approach. In particular, the general degradation of the brain's operations, and the loss of essential neurochemical output, is a result of the symbion feeding off of the chemically-rich human nervous system, a vast network of 100 billion specialized cells. These cells, neurons, transmit signals along neural pathways and provide a virtual tour of reality. These intricate interactions largely determine the behaviour of the life form. An entity jacked into that vital network will necessarily impact behaviour and perception. Any foreign device that interrupts those chemical interactions also will interrupt the actions of a person, and we get this cascade of some degradation.

For example, the depletion of the neurotransmitter acetylcholine leads to compromised memory states, and could be diagnosed as Alzheimer's in an advanced state of disrepair. The depletion is a result of a squid-like vampire affixed to some neural channels. The entity gets comfortable with its steady supply of chemical food (the human body breaks down bulk food into chemicals as well) and continues to make a permanent home in the host's multidimensional body. The symbion has just enough density to eat acetylcholine.

Morgellons is an infectious disease with a mysterious cause and even more mysterious symptoms. People with morgellons have the sensation of parasites moving and biting beneath the skin. Not on the skin. Beneath the skin. Morgellons is a yet unacknowledged disease by the Center for Disease Control and

Prevention in the U.S.A. It is currently under investigation and the CDC does not know the cause. Morgellons sufferers experience muscle and joint pains, disabling fatigue, mental confusion, and short term memory loss. These symptoms easily fit our symbion pathology.

A condition similar to morgellons but without the parasitic itch, is fibromyalgia. It is a disease with an unknown etiology (cause), abnormal pains, migraines, psychological distress, foggy memory, and insomnia. Morgellons and fibromyalgia share many similarities, all of which are likely being caused by either a symbion attachment, or in the case of morgellons, some kind of symbion swarm. More so is the presence of psychological disturbance, especially memory problems.

Memory we know is linked to Alzheimer's and to a neural network interruption. Joint pains is connected to arthritis, yet another serious condition with an unknown cause. Some symbions like to chew on cartilage, ligaments, and even the myelin on pain receptor channels. They attach themselves to the lower back, to hands, to hips, and to necks. Symbion attachments not on the nervous system, but on the joint, cause joint pain and inflammation. If these symbions remain for the longer-term, and as a person ages and loses regenerative abilities, they begin to degenerate the joints.

Symbions are also sentient and extremely childish and negative. Once they lock into the host's thought channels, including probably chemical messages, they begin to inject their evil ideas, ideas which may or may not be perceived by the host. This is where the psychosis originates. The psychosis is not originating from the host, although it will appear that way, rather it is the parasite's thoughts that are colliding with the thoughts of the host.

For example, the host's wife arrives home late from work. The symbion suggests to the host (the husband) that the wife is a part-time prostitute. The late wife gets combined with prostitute and the host fills in the blanks, "My wife is having an affair!" Of course this is news to the wife. But the already irritated and now angry husband might take this argument further, and this scenario may build over weeks and months, even recalling old memories to really stir up the paranoia.

From a reality-based perspective the host is being manipulated by the symbion. I am isolating this discussion somewhat to highlight the influence from the entity. Of course, there can be many other factors involved: side effects of drugs, native disposition of individual, propensity for violence or it may even be the case that the wife *is* having an affair and the host had gained some prophetic powers!

When the western health practitioner assigns a disease as a cause of other symptoms they may be giving the patient a disservice. I'd like to repeat that I am not a doctor and have no medical training whatsoever. I am, on the other hand, a reality scientist who is now making an application of this cosmic knowledge to medicine, chiefly to incurable diseases, because I think it offers a missing link.

The human body is a complex molecular machine and the neurons and glia maintain the highway of signal transmission and reception. It is a very delicate process and a technological agent with its tentacles inside of its nervous system is without a doubt going to antagonize a host's (person's) vital life processes. What is interesting, and key, about quite a number of incurable diseases is the presence of changes in behaviour: depression, anxiety, paranoia, anger, delusions, apathy. This is not only due to the siphoning of neurochemicals, but also due to the symbiotic psychic link to the human brain and the psychological attacks on the host, in order to subdue the host.

Why does a symbion want a depressed and diseased host? Because it wants to feed. Every animal is programmed to forage for its food in a particular way so that it can survive. To survive for the long-term the symbion does not wish to kill its host for that is not its purpose. Symbions want to move into the host for the long-term. This is also why many incurable diseases take 10 or 15 years to manifest. Slowly but surely the symbion siphons off the essential molecular nutrients of the body and without any real awareness to what is happening the individual will mysteriously get sick, the kind of sickness that will battle top medical professionals.

A very important component of hacking a human is the psychological element. The disempowering words, the negative thoughts, the reinforced sadism, the drive to act impulsively, the sudden disappearance of inhibition, the rise in worry, the suicidal thoughts and the removal of life's pleasures — all of these and more seem to be present with symbion attacks. But psychotherapy and going to church may not be enough to counter a truly unique, if not alien, pathogen.

There is no medicine or treatment to remove these pathogens with any sense of permanence, and although some gifted healers can indeed clean them from their body the world is littered with all manner of symbions. Until a proper treatment can be invented, the best thing to do, and the first step, is to understand and accept this plausible scenario, as strange as it sounds. It sounds strange today but hopefully tomorrow it will become increasingly familiar. I'll be the first to admit that decoding new technologies is a tough challenge. I have spent many thousands of hours to reach this stage of awareness and this book of observations and suggestions on how to deal with symbions is the kind of book I wish I'd had some years ago.

Further, the effects of a symbion on an individual is predetermined by the characteristics of the individual. And an individual predisposed to violence will, when fuelled by negativity and destruction, only became more violent, even criminal. A person who is loving and compassionate may, when entrenched in negativity, fall into deep anxiety and worry. So if we compared these two symbion victims we'd get two very distinct set of symptoms, and perhaps even a distinct symbion because a symbion could also adapt its DNA to suit the host.

It is easy to lose medical perspective when dealing with advanced technologies and you really have to pay attention to understand the full extent of the situation. If you are battling symbion effects, and your behaviour is unstable, you may have a misdiagnosis. It is important that you yourself do not jump to any conclusion and to work with a medical professional.

As if these conditions were not enough, we also have to take into account that the symbion is corrupting the cellular data and proteins. It is harming your physiological functions as well and because of this we will see an increase in antibodies or an elevation in cytokines, communicative protein molecules typically found in the immune system. For this reason we will believe that neural plaques and tangles have damaged key neurological centers. There is a physiological, physical, component to this multidimensional infestation.

All of this can be rather overwhelming — an invisible energy, a mysterious onset of disease, a prescription of drugs, an impaired existence. It may be sometime before the human mind can accept some of my assertions, and that is okay. I am introducing a never-before-seen medical illness, an illness that at its fundamental root has an alien parasite that is well beyond the imaging systems of the best medical machines. Find a way to make sense of your own particular situation and you may be able to conquer your illness.

INFLUENZA WARHEADS

On September 26, 1918, up to 50,000 people in Massachusetts had the flu and nearly 200 Bostonians died that day. The Spanish Flu had reached the Boston shore and the deadly disease was spreading throughout the military bases. Nearly all the army camps were under quarantine. It was nearing the end of the 1914 War. The world war would end in about 46 days on November 11, 1918. Nine million combatants would be counted dead. But that would pale in comparison to the 100 million deaths from the flu outbreak.

The 1918 Flu came in two waves. The first wave was in spring and the effects would not last. The second wave, on the other hand, would strike hard, even surprising the medical authorities who were not prepared for a killer influenza. It was a contagious respiratory illness highlighted by fever, chills, muscle aches, fatigue, sore throat, and even pneumonia.

In the United States, the flu virus might cause an average of 30,000 deaths per year, with most people well over 65 years old. Most flu symptoms start 1 to 4 days after the flu virus has entered the body. The 1918 Flu was killing people in less than 48 hours and those people were young, strong, and healthy—a complete contradiction to the typical flu variant. The mortality rate hovered up to nearly 50%.

Even after thorough study of the flu virus and using the best medical equipment available, there is no treatment for the flu. The best action is an outdated vaccine. It is outdated because the virus mutates as it spreads. The vaccine requires months to process and by the time it is administered the vaccine does not match the virus. The 1918 Flu was so deadly that it reminded people of a plague two or three thousand years ago. The early plagues did the same thing—it killed strong and healthy young people. *Flu* author Gina Kolata writes, "The worst were plagues that changed the course of history and spelled doom for societies. They even changed human evolution." She continues, "When everyone else is dying, the resistant people will be the ones who remain to propagate. Their genes will begin to predominate."

The effects of the 1918 Flu basically put an end to army activities. Camps were filled with sick soldiers, the drafts were called off and areas on the US map were quarantined. Over 25% of the US population became ill, but probably 40% of the military got sick. Germany, Austria and Italy, the Central Powers, took a heavier hit than the Allies, France, Britain and Russia. The flu reared its ugly head in the spring of 1918, but it wouldn't be until August when the death tolls would start to rise significantly. The entrance of one of the most deadly diseases ever to strike mankind coincided with the end to World War I. It was even argued that the Allies ended on top because of the ravages from a flu virus.

No matter how you view the Spanish Flu of 1918, there can be no mistake that this was not an infectious respiratory illness killing people in a handful of hours, turning their feet black, filling their lungs full of fluid. In the history of earth, the 1918 Flu, a mostly forgotten epidemic though slightly better remembered than the encephalitis lethargica epidemic that occurred around the same time — and both diseases have no known cause and cure — was a freak of nature. It was more than an anomaly. It was the kind of technological application that coincidentally fits well with a spinning pillar of pathogens, verily a *symbion tornado*. The kind of invisible weapon that is too advanced to be in the hands of mortal men.

To purposely kill 100 million people with nothing more than infectious air is a pretty impressive feat. You have to think about one central aspect of the 1918 conundrum — it has not since reappeared (it might have appeared as the Black Death in the fourteenth century, nearly 600 years before). Pandemics and plagues have been around for centuries. Moses and the Pharaoh of Egypt battled each other with plagues. Long before 1918, plagues and global pandemics were considered godly devices, but even the mysteries of this deadly flu were not enough to convince people that it was stranger than it appeared.

Given a new understanding of incurable diseases, and now having some familiarity with artificially produced symptoms, it is perfectly in the realm of possibility to infect the world using symbion technology. But this technology would have to be very advanced, advanced enough to break through the immune system and to corrupt cells turning the immune system against the body and having the body kill itself. The key would be to compromise the immune system and to corrupt the glia. This is a very advanced technology employed by multidimensional scientists and given the falseness of reality it can only mean that there are some masters who have managed to remain hidden. What they have provided is more evidence of their presence.

My discovery of three synthetic politicians in Washington, DC not only put robot technologies on the table. More importantly I think it revealed three significant fingerprints of some advanced agency, the kind of agency better relegated to science fiction novels. In this case though, the agency was interfering with real lives. They had inserted androids at the highest levels of the US government and were using them to influence the nation's leaders and public policies, thereby controlling society. To control society, they only need to control leadership, but since they could not always put a robot in for President they had robots working as presidential advisers. The android fingerprints convinced me that there was another agency outside of human perception.

The presence of incurables is yet more evidence to support that idea. We live in a fixed biological bubble, verily an ecosystem, and in that bubble we have people afflicted by things which are not only outside of modern medical treatment, but also outside of spirituality, prayer, and good karma. Incurables defy every tool mankind has to offer and they do not afflict two or three individuals. They afflict two or three percent of the population.

An anomaly in the population would be 100 people in 30 million. One hundred people with some strange disease out of thirty million people would be considered an anomaly. When you have 900,000 patients in 30 million afflicted with an incurable disease this is no longer an anomaly. This is evidence.

When 30% of society is obese, this is evidence. When 20% of the population suffers from depression, this is evidence. When 10% of society is on antipsychotics, including teens, this is evidence. When diabetes and Alzheimer's spring out of nowhere, this is evidence. When breast cancer rates, after 50 years of awareness, show growth rather than show decline, this is evidence.

All of it and more is evidence of an advanced kind of technological application at work. An application still outside of human thought and humanity needs to expand its thinking in order to reverse the growth of incurables. We cannot afford to learn to live with all these artificially induced diseases. We need to learn their true cause and to put them all into remission, and eventually to find a permanent cure. Human civilization isn't very far from making all disease extinct, if only medicine is capable of expanding its game play.

Look at the significance of the political map at the time of the Spanish Flu: at the end of the First World War, the Allies were in control and the Central Powers had been defeated. Millions of soldiers were suffering from the flu and could not fight. This technological flu played a significant role in the end of the war. We could say that the flu effectively *ended* the war, but since it struck the members of the Central Powers more severely than the Allies we could say that this was not an accident. We are now describing a very significant geo-political device that can reshape the world map. Either the Allies had good karma or they had a good chess player on some other dimension.

The flu is a highly generalized term since there are many types of flu. The common flu symptoms, as we have said, can be artificially induced with symbion devices. A small swarm of symbions can engulf a person and can entangle their immune system. The symbions only need to break through the immune shield in order to corrupt protein molecules or glia cells to make the illness all that more serious.

The grade of the symbion attachments for flu are of a much lower value than those for Alzheimer's. We know this because the illness is of a much lower value and therefore we can see that there are several grades of symbions. The grade of the symbion is a reflection of not only its complexity but also of its intelligence. An intelligent symbion can be programmed to cripple a target for the long term. It can usher in arthritis and it can create Lou Gehrig's. It depends on the complexity and the complexity depends on the creator.

What has been implicit in our discussion is the presence of an invisible hand behind the evolution of humanity. That there is some unknown agency influencing, even determining, the course of human history, and in the case of plagues and deadly outbreaks we can be assured that the geo-political map has changed hands. This must necessarily be according to a plan. And the chess board of earth is not a free-for-all. There are rules.

If there weren't rules why 97% of the world would be afflicted with an incurable. The fact that only about 3% are afflicted tells us that there are some ground rules. Only so many people can be diseased, only so many can be killed off, only so many can be depressed at any one time. People might think of it as luck but really it's a game and if there were no ground rules, there would be no earth. It would be a ghost planet.

Now that we have established the possibility of a technology designed to cripple millions of people with incurable diseases we are no longer able to believe in all of life's mysteries. We now have to face the fact that a hidden agency has been shaping society. While this agency may have many historical names, I am not so eager to give it a name with any negative connotation because we really don't know what we are dealing with yet.

After I discovered the androids in Washington, after I was convinced by my observations and evidence, I could not help to conclude that those androids were built by some advanced scientific agency. I did speculate that with at least one of the androids, chiefly the female, that she could be the embodiment of one of those master agents. A chief master agent could be inhabiting her body for prolonged periods at a time and in doing so it meant that this master agent did not have its own physical form in this world. It had to borrow a form and that form was one which they created some years earlier.

Now, we have the case of something else. We have the presence of symbions and these symbions are inducing incurable disease. While these incurables are keeping the pharmaceuticals profitable they are at the same time destroying lives and families. This kind of book offers a kind of redemption from centuries of suffering. That if this knowledge can be properly applied, rather than feared and forgotten, if this material can be implemented even by the few then it means that the rate of incurables can be reduced, and over the years it is possible to virtually remove these incurable diseases. There is no immediate cure. But there is a cause.

The flu is of particular interest because of its prevalence. Even it is not the killer flu of 1918 or the H1N1 of 2009 (a cryptic variant), the flu is still an ongoing concern. It is a seasonal infection that has less to do with biology than with technology. At the very least, through our understanding of symbions we can cure the flu, and even colds for that matter. We can also revisit events like the Spanish Flu epidemic to gain new insights into how the world is shaped.

In my view, the flu is an artificial illness. We not only can we free ourselves from the ravages of the flu, more so, we can reduce the symptoms without drugs. If we can overcome the flu we can work our way to overcoming more serious diseases.

CAUSING CURES

The application of reality science on medically-recognized incurable diseases is an opportunity to alleviate common symptoms with a possibility of finding an actual cure. The diagnosis of any serious illness is not to be taken lightly and has come about from clinical observations and rigorous tests. We can in no way dismiss the clinical diagnosis. In fact we are relying now on the diagnosis as a platform with which to apply an unscientific application and to deal with a completely new multidimensional cause, the negatively-charged symbion.

My assessment of the symbiotic program is based on my firsthand experience with its devastating effects and is further supported by my extensive observations in daily life. When this unique understanding was matched with a specific set of incurable diseases, using my own unorthodox methodology, I discovered an amazing correlation between symptoms of disease and symptoms of symbion attachments. That now presented an entirely unique and plausible cause for diseases which were established to have no cause. The appearance of a cause, even if invisible and difficult to detect, is also the discovery of a possible cure. If there is a cause, there is a cure.

The alternative discussions on medical system origins present us with a whole new substrate of medicine that is plausible paranormal exercise and not necessarily scientifically worthy. While I tried my best not to diminish the significance of an incurable disease, I also stated that the cause of at least some of these mysterious diseases could be attributed to an attached symbion pathogen. There was no known cause or cure because the cause has a multidimensional symbiotic organism that fed off of human chemistry.

There is no clinical study of symbions that I am aware of (plus the equipment for proper observations are not invented yet), although there are paranormal studies that may be a result of symbionic organisms. There are a reliable number of medical symptoms of each disease that, rather than a result from a mystery, could have resulted from an advanced parasite embedded into the nervous system.

Certainly it is plausible to suggest that a device that can access certain parts of a human anatomy could compromise the health of an individual. Given that this may be one of the few extensive discussions, in public anyway, on a very provocative topic, and trusting that—my experiences and observations are accurate enough, we can at least assume that this work can be further developed in the months and years to come.

Medical doctors are trained to heal their patient's ailments, and specialists are called upon to resolve health issues in highly socialized areas, but doctors are not routinely educated on paranormal applications. To most orthodox practitioners many of the medical treatments of today are a result of improvement over supernatural diagnoses and magic potions. So there isn't any risk to revert back to nineteenth century experimental medicine. By the same token, I have directly experienced symbions for several years (that I was consciously aware of) and have gone through many, if not more, of the symptoms associated with incurable diseases. Because of my personalized therapeutic approach I have, so far, avoided the onset of a serious illness.

In primitive medicines of the nineteenth century what I have discussed here would be considered paranormal and supernatural experiences which may or may not include neuropsychological imbalances and/or psychiatric need. Both Freud and Jung stood out as physicians because they were able to create a new paradigm of diagnosis, and they did so by inventing a more humane treatment. Look at Jung's interaction with the disassociated schizophrenic at one of the asylums. Jung kept an open mind and four years later the strange things about the origins of the wind was corroborated in an ancient Egyptian spell.

What does it really mean when the knowledge inside the mind of a mentally ill man has some ancient validity, the kind of validity that defies logic and coincidence? That is what I think Jung was acknowledging because how sick can this man be if he knew about Egyptian magic. This was further of interest to Jung who originally intended to be an Egyptologist so he knew full well of the advanced culture of the pharaohs, the same architects of the pyramids. How can a man with schizophrenia (*dementia praecox* in those days), verily a crazy person, how can he know about this kind of advanced knowledge?

We sort of have an explanation for this phenomenon, don't we? Because we have some new understandings of the brain. In reality medicine, the speed of the neural pathways in the brain can determine the level of access to the matrix of reality. These pathways we assume to be chiefly axons and axons are insulated with myelin and glia. In order to speed up the electrical signals shooting through the axons we need to have better insulation; otherwise, there is a short-circuit. You can't race a Ferrari down a dirt road. You need a properly paved, clean, and walled race track. People with schizophrenia must have some very good race tracks that allow their brains to hit top speed and in reaching top speed they can peer outside of reality. They can look back 5,000 years to ancient Egypt perhaps.

You know, what we are doing is providing some additional substance to the psychic phenomena. That if the neural circuits were advanced enough and if the myelin insulation was thick enough then some brains could do amazing things. But there is a catch — these brains often crash and when they crash these people end up in mental hospitals. We also know something else, don't we? We know that symbions (being parasites) like to chew on glia and myelin. The demyelination of a superior brain could lead to distortions in thinking, chemical leaks, hallucinations, delusions, and psychotic episodes: all of which would be given some psychiatric label (eg paranoid schizophrenia).

Psychoanalysis in particular was less of a treatment than some kind of debugging tool. A person's inner machine had become corrupted, the processors were producing invalid results and psychotherapy was applied to relink specific memories to the right neurological channels. Of course I am saying this based on my understanding of the situation. Each person cannot be so easily explained. But it makes sense. If these parasites are eating away at the chemicals and circuitry of the person's brain, in some ways it is shorting out the circuitry and causing power outages. This would be no different than having an 8-year old kid with a tool box playing with the fuse box to your home, only that your home's electrical system doesn't regenerate half as well as the nervous system.

I think Freud and Jung played a pivotal role in redirecting the fate of humanity. Instead of heading into commercialized psychosurgery and electro-convulsive shock therapy, psychiatry became equipped to apply a more humanistic touch. We see the results 130 years later — today's children with ADHD aren't being lobotomized and having portions of their brains removed. It doesn't matter that we haven't reached my level of discussion, what matters is that humans with mental imbalances are being treated more humanely than they would have if Freud and Jung hadn't been teaching their psychoanalytical doctrines. Imagine if nations were still sterilizing mentally ill people as they did in the 1930s and those advanced genes weren't getting passed on. We might've seen the disappearance of a certain magical class of citizens.

The situation isn't perfect today. Handing out antidepressants to children isn't the way forward but it is better than a) the kid never being born, or, b) the kid having chunks of his brain removed. The chief problems with Freud, Jung, et al is that they were not able to make the next leap in logic. And I have only been able to make the next leap because of the work they started. All of them. All of these related scientists and physicians; because of them I am able to identify a possible cure to the most perplexing diseases on the planet.

I must insist that my symptoms are being primarily caused by a range of symbion agents, and if these symptoms are consistent with certain incurables then it could only be the case that there is an association between symbions and incurables. Yet, unlike modern clinical observations, my symbions cannot be measured with any known medical equipment and are therefore subject to severe scientific scrutiny.

I can justify that my theory is much more than a theory because I am able to negate the effects of a symbiote, and at the same time, remove the symptoms. The symptomatic relief reinforces the association between these invisible entities and an incurable disease. I truly feel that the symbions present a plausible curative effect for some persons afflicted with life-changing illnesses, and, at the very minimum, can likely provide some symptomatic relief since we are invariably focused on the nervous system and the neurological components in particular. The better we understand how the brain works the better we are able to determine what kind of symbion is attached and, quite possibly, what it is programmed to do. By understanding the type of symbion, and even the predisposition of the host, we are able to figure out ways to either remove it or to counter its chemical takeover.

If the corruption of proteins in the nervous system, or even in specific neurological structures like the basal ganglia and substantia nigra, activates antibodies that cannot distinguish between a foreign agent and a normal protein then the antibodies will end up attacking aspects of the host, and the physiological degradation will lead to a batch of

242

symptoms. As the symbion continues to hack the host's operation centers the immune system continues to degrade the health of the individual. The faster an intervention the less likely any permanent damage will take place as a result of the attachment and the more likely a remission and a cure will take place.

On the surface it might seem I am attributing a single cause to a disease. I am not. The cause of the disease is a multi-tentacle semi-intelligent organism/agent that is programmed to hack the central processing center of the human. So we are discussing multiple attacks to the headquarters of the individual and this is how it can take over a complex carbon-based life form (ie human body).

It is not in the scope of this book to treat the cause of diseases, although in some areas suggested treatments were made. Because of disease complexity and due to such a provocative medical situation any treatment must include a comprehensive educational analysis of what exactly we are dealing with; otherwise, people will easily become overwhelmed and will still get sick (flare ups).

This must include the synthetic nature of life, and, expectedly, this aspect will prove quite a challenge for orthodox minds

It is very clear from my personal experience that these symbiotic entities need to gain a psychological dominance in order to have any substantial influence. If the host simply is able to refuse any of the negative propaganda or wild ideas then the symbion will not be allowed further control. It will then sit dormant or may even die off due to a lack of chemical foods. As well, a person who is keen on a healthy lifestyle may be able to remove the symbion just by maintaining a clear and healthy lifestyle, especially one with an exceptional frequency of vibration. Symbions prefer low frequency vehicles and weak-minded hosts, and a high frequency person is harder to hack. That does not stop from trying especially when they were created for that very purpose.

The symbion device is both a naturally existing device and an artificially created device. They are often created by reality programmers (sorcerers) and used to subdue or remove disliked persons. They are also attracted by the host to serve specific actions (by way of attraction and intention). For example, some people who expect a headache, may welcome a symbion in order to manifest their desired outcome. The types of symbions can be quite a few. In this book I have only addressed the introductory versions, and even these are sufficient enough to cause incurable illness, even death.

Introducing a negatively charged multidimensional pathogen could lead people to allocate them in the paranormal box and intentionally avoiding a primordial tool used in reality planes of existence. Basically, we may throw away the only real chance to cure of slate of previously incurable diseases and will turn away from a technological medicine primed for an advanced future. If my experience is anything to go by, and I think it is, then at the very least I have identified a symptomatic cause that could alleviate sufferer's symptoms and would reduce the burden on healthcare systems. Moreover, if I am accurate and can develop more advanced reality medical techniques then it is within the realm of possibility that I have discovered the path to the end of disease. And that is worthy thinking about.

SOME WAYS TO APPROACH ILLNESS AND DISEASE

A NEW APPROACH TO DISEASE

This knowledge and thinking provided in this book is without a doubt unorthodox. It is also not scientifically proven. If I have learned anything from my work, it is the fact that conventional science cannot explain everything. It can only explain some things. The presence of incurable disease alone proves my point— science cannot identify cause or cure of a number of diseases. This does not mean that the diseases do not exist. Quite the contrary, the lack of scientific explanation means that scientific thinking has not kept up with existential evolution. More specifically, since my work has profoundly been focused on manufactured realities, scientific theories have not kept up with humanity's interaction with this plane of existence.

A plane of existence is like a computer system. As the processor speeds up, the hard drive gets bigger, the monitor gets sharper, and the box gets smaller. It works as a system because all the software developers and hardware manufacturers work in tandem to improve the system. We do not see in the information technology industry a 200-pound computer running the latest Intel microprocessor. In fact, we see quite the opposite, don't we? We see a faster processor inside of a better-designed box, such as the recent introduction of tablet computers. These are powerful handheld computing and communication devices.

The real world is not as harmonious as the computer world. In the real world we have twenty-third century computers alongside war, religion, and nineteenth century science. Our automobiles primarily use the internal combustion engine and run on gasoline, these technologies are over 100 years old. Christianity was invented 1,700 years ago, at a time when the idea of software could not exist alongside an all powerful deity. And our homes are powered by electricity, an artefact of Tesla, Edison, and Westinghouse, among other contemporaries. The electrical lighting in our homes and work places are the remnants of Edison's Pearl Street Station. It was on Pearl Street where the first central power station was located in America. In

1882 about 400 lamps in 85 homes were lit by electricity. One hundred and thirty years later we are still using electrical power stations to light our lamps and power our TVs.

When we add incurable diseases into the picture, we get a world that is anything but harmonious. Earth is not in harmony because all of our thoughts are not in harmony. Reality medicine allows us a small chance to improve one area of thought, health. But to be successful in applying this healing application we have to rethink how we approach illness and disease. We have to incorporate some new ideas and thinking into regeneration and recuperation. The better we apply these new medical technologies the more likely a cure can be found. It won't happen right away because we will be amateurs for a good long while. Some of us will have innate abilities to think in these terms and may have always known principles in synthetic healing without ever recognizing it.

The Flu (Influenza)

The seasonal flu has been around for centuries. Doctors advise rest, fluids, good grooming, medication, and vaccinations. Millions of people will get the flu every year. It lasts about a week. It is likely to hit someone more than once. A few might die from complications. A few might only have it a few days. A few will rarely get the flu.

Armed now with some new medical thinking, we can approach the flu from a whole new level. To start off we can transcribe the flu, an aerosol-virus (it can travel through the air), into a kind of symbion-based pathogen. Imagine that the all-mysterious influenza is in fact the result of a symbion attack on the immune system. If the immune system is defeated and the symbion is able to enter the metabolic structures then a viral attack is a likely result. To the extent that the immune system is compromised we can estimate the severity of the flu on the person. In other words, there is no single type of illness. The illness is a result of immunity. The strength of the immunity is dependent on the strength of the symbion.

Now I am talking about the seasonal flu, mostly. There is the other kind of flu strain, the Spanish flu and the Bird flu as examples. While these pandemics can have symbion participation the root of the viral attack is likely some weaponized biological agent. The two of them work hand in hand, the biological agent weakens the human immune system on the physical level while the technological device is able to attach itself to the nervous system.

We can hear the traces of the oncoming flu by the number of sniffles at the office or in the classroom. The sniffles indicate the immune system at work. As soon as we notice these indicators — people sniffling, friends calling in sick, sneezing, coughing, fevers, feeling run down, and the other standard flu indicators — we should prepare our minds to improve our immune system. We should improve our diets to strengthen our immune systems. And now we should do daily bodily cleansing of symbions.

Cleansing the body of symbion attachments can be quite complex. Some of them may have been there for quite some time as we will see in addictions. Usually, flu-related symptoms indicate newer symbion attacks. It is important to prevent their attachments because they could wreak internal havoc on the body in the years to come. One thing that symbions (and other negative entities) do not like is water, especially sea water and river water. Taking a daily hot bath is an ideal technique to cleanse some of these pathogens from your multidimensional system. You can add sea salt for an added boost. Check with your health food store or practitioner on essential oils you can add to your bath. The daily bath allows you a chance to correct any imbalance and to dissolve their attachments. Of course, hot baths (even showers) are best before any infection symptoms have begun. Once you have fever and coughs it will be much harder to remove them for they have attached themselves. In any case, you shouldn't worry. You have been doing this for your entire life only now you have some new approaches. Your immune system is very advanced and boosting your own defences is an excellent strategy.

What I am essentially saying, but haven't said clearly, is that there is no such thing as the flu. The flu is the result of a technological pathogen. It is not a mysterious illness that happens seasonally. This is like telling adults that Santa Claus is real only in December. What is the case though is that periodically there are millions of symbions floating through the air. Let's put aside the biological agents added by malevolent agencies and focus on the naturalistic flu.

We know that millions of people each year for a good many years get sick and this sickness is called the flu. It all appears to be normal. We accept it. I am saying that there is no such thing as the flu. Well, if each person required one symbion, just one, and say 10 million people got the flu in September then that means there are at minimum 10 million symbions. Where are the 10 million symbions coming from?

It is an important question and one that we haven't specifically talked about. The symbions are coming from the earth. How is that possible? Aren't symbions generated by malicious agents? Yes, but symbion technologies did not originate from these malicious groups. In fact, the creation of symbions must necessarily be created from the reality architecture. A symbion cannot exist outside of the reality and in this case they have a limited dimensional range. People who have a very high vibration and a potent immune system naturally dissolve symbions, even by the hundreds. These people are unlikely to get the flu unless they have weakened their immune system somehow (eg partying, poor nutrition, overwork).

Why would the earth periodically release these technological pathogens? Because these pathogens are also programs and these programs contain new reality codes. Remember that a symbion can cause disease because it latches itself onto the neurological system and it hacks into the DNA and reprograms the manufacture of proteins. The mutated proteins reprogram the rest of the DNA and this eventually leads to a weakness and then a disease. The process can be slow or fast according to the human defence and human awareness. The greater the human awareness the greater the defence. (Reading this book has already improved your resistance to these (and other) pathogens, something you may or may not be aware of for a while.)

What is fundamentally true is the fact that reality uses these existential programs (symbions) to upgrade the system and it is periodically upgrading the system to such an extent that your eyes cannot see it ever taking place. What our conventional scientists have done is to dwindle down a very advanced reality protocol into some kind of illness. See, modern medicine is telling everyone that they need medication and vaccination to battle the flu virus. The flu is an enemy in the mind of the doctor. That once again goes back to what we discussed about nineteenth century science. Reality-based medicine has the opposite view. It says that we are living inside of a progressive plane of existence and that it periodically must upgrade the existential software. One of the methods the planet uses to upgrade itself is by releasing these advanced apps.

The programming charge they contain will ensure that each citizen is up-to-date. The people who are the most out-dated and have the oldest software codes usually need a bigger download and therefore get "sick." But it's not as much a "sickness" as much as it is an "upgrade." What conventional wisdom says is an attack and an illness is not the case with reality wisdom which says the seasonal flu is more akin to a seasonal DNA upgrade.

The more up-to-date your internal systems are the less likely that a flu will hit you. A properly functioning immune system will regularly upgrade itself from using the environmental programs. These kinds of people are typically conscious of what they eat, they exercise regularly, and they are careful not to overdo any activity, including thinking. A person who rarely gets sick is a person who is listening to their body and aware of the reality effects at the subconscious level. If you are one of these people keep doing what you are doing. If you are the opposite, if you get really sick during flu season, then your system could be out of sync with reality or it could have some genetic weaknesses.

You can try to improve these conditions by identifying exactly what is going on. Talking to an alternative doctor or studying alternative

257

health may be a way to help you toward better health. Don't be afraid of the flu. It is not the flu. It might just be a system upgrade.

At the very least you should pay closer attention to your immune system as the symbions wear down your defences. This is natural so you have to counter that with additional care and attention. The key is to reinterpret a disease as a technological protocol. It assumes that you can accept the fact that reality is artificially constructed. Take your time and work within your own set of limitations.

In any case, avoid jumping to extremes because they don't last and they can cause harm to your system. Slowly retrain your thinking to move away from illness to improvement. Should you notice a new flu strain turning into a pandemic then that may be one that is being artificially induced by some malicious group. If there are weaponized biological agents involved be extra careful. In no time flat, the system upgrade will be done and you'll be up-to-date until next time.

Depression

If depression is a result of an attachment from a negatively programmed being then the cure is not necessarily found in an antidepressant. A pharmaceutical drug may give your own system a necessary boost, but as well if you are depressed by a symbion and you take a drug to raise certain neurochemicals then the symbion will likely feed off of those chemicals and it will further attach itself to your nervous system. The drugs you take can lead to making the symbion stronger and a strong symbion will stay in your system for the long term. Mild depression could morph into chronic depression.

If we know that these symbions may be present, assuming that we do not have a genetic deformity or other malady, then to cure ourselves of depression we need to weaken the symbion's effects on our nervous system. We pay close attention to our health, diets, exercise, frame of mind, and lifestyle. We take natural supplements and we ask nutrition experts for their advice. If the symbions have penetrated our defences deep enough then this could lead to suicidal thoughts. It doesn't take much to drive a depressed person into having suicidal thoughts. But we now know that if depression is created by an attack from a multidimensional entity then we know that it is not because we are bad people.

Depressed people may focus on certain negative aspects of their lives, but that is what the symbion is influencing your thoughts to focus on. They are coordinating your sensory flow and that flow is laced with negative memories. You are not a bad person because you have these negative experiences. We all have negative experiences (eg failures, embarrassments, imperfections, rejections). It is when you focus on those negative memories too much that you become severely depressed but that is the result of an advanced sensory manipulator. You are very likely under attack so you should try not to focus on those negative memories.

Every time the symbion stimulates your negative memories you have to consciously think of positive memories. You have to avoid intensifying any negative experience and to put things into perspective. At the same time you should be tending to your body so as to reduce these symbions. If you do not believe those negative memories and you reject the symbion's control mechanisms then you are starving these pathogens. Without your feeding they become weak, their attachments loosen and they are easier to remove. Their attachments will dissolve sooner than you think.

If you believe those negative memories and you start to magnify them then you feed the symbion and then you can become more depressed and suicidal. You may do something stupid. You may feel like causing harm to yourself. I have had these attacks and quite often is the case, the symbions, once they get deeply attached, they want me to harm my body. They want me to cause physical damage on myself.

If they could not get me to harm myself then they wanted me to act wildly causing me to have an accident. If I was using a pair of scissors they tried to influence me to act with carelessness and that carelessness would lead to an accidental cut. The cut would lead me to release some emotion, say anger, and the release of that emotion indicated a release of a neurochemical and that is what they wanted. They need to eat to stay alive. They don't care about you. They want to influence you to release more neurochemicals.

The phase of suicide is so extreme is so rich in neurotransmitter activity that it is like a gigantic symbion buffet. If the symbion was created by some malicious agent that agent may also share some of your energy in your moment of crisis. Some dark agents (eg sorcerers) feed off of this suicidal energy, like a drug, and they get a kick out of driving people into these dark shadows. If you realize that you are being attacked and manipulated then you owe it to yourself to put up a defence. That defence includes staying calm and rational. If you get angry you feed them. If you stay calm you stay in control. And you want to stay in control.

In reality-based medicine, depression is the symptom of a symbion attachment and severe depression is a result of either a more advanced symbion or a group of symbions. The chemical imbalance is not because a person is malfunctioning, which is the conventional interpretation, rather there is a foreign agent that is interfering with the natural neurological processes. To cure yourself of depression you need to realize that you are not necessarily malfunctioning. Secondly, you need to realize that you could have a symbion attachment that is interfering with your conscious life. And thirdly you need you to proactively remove or reduce the effects of this multidimensional symbiote.

We are not always able to correct our living situations. We may be living in a very difficult family environment or we may need certain negativistic friends (or bosses). So the remedy isn't always immediately available. The best you can do is to compensate for your miserable life. Find things that make you smile. Listen to certain kinds of music or spend time with people you love. Life is not all roses and as you get older it becomes even more thorny, even hostile, so sometimes you have to learn to manage the depressive feelings (with as few substances as possible) rather than to find a permanent cure.

I have seen situations where a mass of symbions were removed from a person and within hours a new set of symbions had attached themselves to the individual. This kind of person can spend 24 hours a day removing symbions and not spend anytime dedicated to their lives or they can learn to manage these entities and to live in such a way as to maintain a certain amount of dignity. It is unlikely that you can remove serious disease-related symbions at this stage. This may urge you to study artificial causes further so that in time you can master this aspect of your life. Again, the key is always to realize that your depression is the result of symbion interference and not because you are malfunctioning. Maintain a positive stream of thinking for as many hours of the day as you can. This is not to be an entertainer and not to be in excess, just turn your mental voltage far enough to enter the zone of positivity and don't allow anything to bring you down. And if you can get rid of certain negative influences, try to do so.

Addiction

What if you cannot become an addict? What would it mean if I said that within the same person, the individual and the addict are two separate entities? If an addict, any kind of addict, is obsessed with a particular form of pleasure (sex, drug, alcohol, gambling, lying, violence, shopping, pain, porn, painkillers) then it should be the case that a symbion entity is involved. In the case of addiction, there is usually more than one symbion present and they have some kind of exchange agreement between them so that there are fresh ones coming to replace the older ones. Why are they there on the person's multidimensional body? They want a joyride. They want a joyride and the human host is ignorant of their presence; for if the host was aware of symbions why they would realize that they are being used by simple-minded creatures. They are not only being used but they are being consumed. Their life force is being consumed and they are so wrapped up in their pleasure that they cannot put things in perspective.

Additionally, there can be at times even larger symbion entities that have literally wrapped themselves around the soul of the individual. Again, no external agency can gain such an access to your internal systems unless you gave it permission. But they are very cunning. They know how to gain your consent. They will ask you if you want pleasure. If you agree then you have given permission. They did not specify the pleasure and addiction is pleasurable, and ultimately very damaging to your life and family. If you do not agree with pleasure they will suggest that you will meet more people and perhaps find someone to love you, and who doesn't want that? These sentient symbiotes will continue to wear away at your psychological defences, even attacking you when you are under stress or emotionally upset, until they get the permission they want. And once they get their foot in the door they want to fully dominate you.

Rehab cannot succeed unless the demons are conquered. The demons may lay quiet while the addict stays at rehab, or they may even just remove themselves so that the addict can appear to be more honest, but once the person feels better they find their way back into their mind. The person, unaware, allows them to attach and the addict soon enough falls off the wagon. It's that little voice that is always there when the temptation begins. Doesn't matter if it's little boys or a bottle of booze, that little voice encourages the reformed addict: "Just a little touch, just a little sip, you earned it, you deserve a little bit of pleasure, you're not a monk."

These voices are not the internal voices of the person. This is a hard part to explain to rationally minded people. These are the voices of symbions. The symbions are hooked into the nervous system and so when they speak it is telepathic. Well, they are jacked into the native communications system of the person. It's very straight-forward for them and they have an agenda — they need to get those brain chemicals moving and they need to get this reformed addict on their drug of choice. Whatever it takes to get the neurons flowing. As far as the symbions go, it doesn't matter if a person gambles, watches porn, molests kids, or robs banks — what they want are those molecular exchanges to take place.

Recovery from addiction begins with a choice. The choice comes from realizing that you are an addict. In my unprofessional view, an addiction is present when there is excess and that excess is unproductive, damaging, negative, and bad for your health and family. If you are addicted to your job, well, we could argue that it's productive. If you are shooting heroin, there's no argument — it's not good for you and a basic waste of time. Addictions could also be said to be complete wastes of time. Watching online porn for four hours is a waste of time. Sure, you might argue it's pleasurable, but I will argue that you are watching online porn because of symbion attachments and that means they are making a fool of you. They are taking the pleasure from you and wasting your life. And when they have consumed your life they will find some other victim.

If you are the type of person who doesn't like being taken advantage of and can see a con before it happens, then this is the biggest con job of them all. Simple-minded demons have conned you into letting them suck the life out of you so that they can have a joyride. And once they get you hooked, you'll never remember them at the helm. I find it sad to see people addicted because I can see that they are being remote controlled by some very low life forms. All it takes is for the addict to say, "Enough is enough." Then to go cold turkey and to realize they don't need whatever they've been fooled to take. They've been fooled to take it like Pavlov's dog.

Once they resist and break the agreement with the symbions, the symbions have to detach. But the key here is to break the majority of the agreements. There is more than one. There can be many agreements. The addict has to search their troubled memory and to figure out where it all started and then to slowly clear it out. The longer they have been hacked the longer the recovery period. If the recovering addict rushes it there can be more problems. It all starts with a decision to live a better life and there's no turning back no matter what.

Neurodegenerative Disease

Alzheimer's, Parkinson's, Multiple Sclerosis, and all the other neurodegenerative diseases take many years of degeneration in order to reach disease status. The diseases set in because of a lack of certain neurochemicals, damage to certain neuronal areas, and the presence of certain mutated proteins, among many other compounds and conditions. The symbions in this case are tapped into those neurotransmitter pathways and are zapping away those chemicals. They are locked onto the myelin sheathing and are eating away at it and as the electricity passes through the unmyelinated axons there is a loss in voltage. There is probably also an electrical leak. That then causes damage to other glial cells. Chronic dopamine shortage leads to Parkinson-like symptoms, perhaps even bouts of catatonia, but all of this is just the intermediary phases. The real damage has yet to reveal itself.

Slowly, over the years the forgetfulness and the palsy form after the neurons have been sufficiently damaged. And it can take years to properly diagnose a neurodegenerative disease. The body, at the same time, is regenerating. When there is damage in the brain the glial cells get to work to repair the damage. The symptoms seem to appear and then seem to disappear. For progressive conditions, the patient gets increasingly worse until they get the diagnosis and by then it is too late. The damage has been done.

Again, my argument remains the same. Among a number of possibilities, the symbions can create all the necessary damage. The lack of human awareness allows this situation to continue. If the person was aware of multidimensional symbiotes then they could learn ways to remedy the damage done by these creatures. The body is very powerful. The glia in particular seem to have an immense ability to repair neurons and to restore harmony in the neurological system. A proper regeneration requires an understanding of both symbions and neurology. As soon as the patient starts taking drugs, the damage is compounded and the person's recovery chance is compromised.

You can prevent the onset of neurodegenerative disease by paying attention to the common symptoms of these incurable illnesses. If you notice the symptoms appearing and disappearing, in a significant pattern, then you can deduce that there are symbions present and you can take early action to remedy them. Unfortunately, no one expects to get an incurable disease and so therefore don't bother to look and are unlikely to know the symptoms. Awareness is a powerful weapon because your awareness of something has a profound impact on your molecular operations. Awareness and understanding allow the genes to do their job properly and that in itself is very good preventive medicine. Sadly, we live in a world that is wholly unaware of the concepts of reality thinking and that puts a lot more people at risk then necessary.

If you or your loved one is suffering from an incurable disease — and they are not familiar with reality-based medical concepts — then it is likely the case of a long period of ignorance or reliance on conventional medicine. Conventional medicine works for bruises and acute illnesses like aneurysms. But when it comes to incurable disease, neither the specialist nor the pharmacist can cure you. You have to work slowly to adopt some of the concepts in this book.

For those who have never thought this way they will need a period of time to get educated and a period of time to adopt a new approach to illness. Most of the time the doctor has convinced the patient that the disease has no cure and that they need some indefinite medicine. Synthetic healing, as you can see, requires a completely different approach. It assumes that the body is infinitely powerful and it understands that there are multidimensional threats that can create disease.

Mental Illness

Mental illness is a medical quagmire. Not only is there no cure for mental illness, there are people's lives involved. Mental illness symptoms can be very serious and difficult to handle. Resolving clinical observations of mentally ill patients with reality-based medical principles is not the intent here. Patients suffering from extreme conditions need proper hospital and medical care. Reality medicine is better applied to people before they have a psychotic episode and after they've had one. For example, after a seizure the patient can learn to calm down faster and to avoid any serious convulsions or unconsciousness simply by understanding the technological threats in the environment.

If we now are realizing that a sentient symbiote is attached to our minds and we are having hallucinations and hearing delusions then we have a chance to separate the truth from symbiotic fiction. If we understand what the truth is, by understanding ourselves, then we can separate the delusions being invented by the attached symbions. Hallucinations are easy to come about when the symbions can influence our visual networks and they can also distort our external lenses to see whatever we want.

Recall that the symbion is an external agent that can also tap into our neurological networks; therefore, they can distort our external visual fields, say by blocking our peripheral vision or by reversing letters and numbers we see, and they can influence the flow of information in our brains. So they can interrupt the memory signals and dial up an old love interest and they can distort the visual signals and project that love interest in plain sight. We will actually see what has been drummed up from our memory.

If our memories were romantic we would have some dreamy hallucination. We might see Jesus and become super religious. And the voice inside our head might even be interpreted as Jesus and Jesus will begin a conversation with us. He may even tell us what to do later on and he may not make sense. But because all of our key internal neurological channels are activated, all of this appears real and true.

We will tell people that we saw Jesus or that we saw a ghost of a loved one. Worse, this situation can turn ugly when there are traumatic memories combined with someone we love. A traumatic experience could be combined with a wife and that could spur us into a psychotic episode whereby we beat our wife for no reason whatsoever.

Once the mind is even partially controlled, it can be corrupted. Any idea can be mixed into the person's mind and this will fundamentally alter their thinking. It will rewire their brain. It can turn an innocent man into a criminal. It can send a rational scientist into a fit of delusional rage. People can lose their careers, families, and lives. A person might chop down an old tree just because Jesus told them to do it. Who is Jesus? Why he's the mental projection that the symbionic entity has constructed. It is hard to explain all the ways a symbion can create mental illness because it also assumes that these creatures are far more capable than we think.

After many personal tests and observations, I can say that the symbion indeed can control key neuronal channels, even multiple channels, and can manifest almost any schizoid environment. After enough of these distortions and cross wires the brain can become wired for mental illness because it no longer runs properly. Medicating a person who is under symbion attack will only make the person worse. If after the symbions are reduced and removed the person still requires medication then that is a much better initiative. There are many people today with a very powerful reservoir of neurochemicals but they take little responsibility for their gifts. A person who needs to recover has to want to recover. A person in denial cannot benefit from reality-based treatment because it requires the willingness of the patient.

Headaches and Migraines

A symbion on the external body, or even on the aura, can create the feelings of a headache. A series of symbions could create a migraine. As well, a symbion with a tentacle in a certain area of your brain can also be experienced as a severe headache. But none of these are headaches and while pain medication will help, so too will exercise and a hot bath. Headaches usually are temporary as the body burns off the negative entities. If the headache is prolonged then some remedy is required: some rest, a hot shower and some exercise. (There can be many reasons for a migraine, some of them can be serious. If it seems serious then consult a physician. Only people who understand their body should do self-diagnosis.)

BIBLIOGRAPHY

Bazil, Carl W., *Living Well with Epilepsy and Other Seizure Disorders*, New York, NY, Harper Collins, 2004.

Breger, Louis, *Freud: Darkness in the Midst of Vision*, John Wiley & Sons, 2000.

Carter, Rita, *The Human Brain Book*, Great Britain, Dorling Kindersley, 2009.

Dawkins, Richard, *The Blind Watchmaker*, London, England, Penguin Books, 2006.

Devinsky, Orrin, *Epilepsy: Patient and Family Guide*, New York, NY, Demos Medical Publishing, 2008.

Doraiswamy, P. Murali, Gwyther, Lisa P., *The Alzheimer's Action Plan: The Expert's Guide to the Best Diagnosis and Treatment for Memory Problems*, New York, NY, St. Martin's Press, 2008.

Fields, R. Douglas, *The Other Brain: From Dementia to Schizophrenia, How New Discoveries about the Brain are Revolutionizing Medicine and Science*, New York, NY, Simon & Schuster, 2009.

Gorman, Jack M., *The Essential Guide to Psychiatric Drugs* (4th ed), New York, NY, St. Martin's Press, 2007.

Gray, Henry, Edited by Pick, T. Pickering, Howden, Robert, *Gray's Anatomy*, London, England, Chancellor Press, 1985.

Jones, Ernest, *The Life and Work of Sigmund Freud: Volume 3*, New York, NY, Basic Books, 1957.

Kandel, Eric R., *In Search of Memory: The Emergence of a New Science of Mind*, New York, NY, WW Norton & Company, 2006.

Kolata, Gina, *Flu: The Story of the Great Influenza Pandemic of 1918 and the Search for the Virus that Caused It*, New York, Farrar, Straus and Giroux, 1999.

Kushner, Howard I., *A Cursing Brain?: The Histories of Tourette Syndrome*, London, England, Harvard University Press, 1999.

Lachman, Gary, *Jung the Mystic: The Esoteric Dimensions of Carl Jung's Life and Teachings,* Jeremy P. Tarcher/Penguin, 2010.

Lahita, Robert G., Phillips, Robert H., *Lupus Q&A: Everything You Need to Know*, New York, NY, Avery, 2004.

LeDoux, Joseph, *Synaptic Self: How Our Brains Become Who We Are*, New York, NY, Viking, 2002.

Machoian, Lisa, *The Disappearing Girl: Learning the Language of Teenage Depression*, London, England, Penguin Books, 2005.

Marion, Robert, *Genetic Rounds: A Doctor's Encounters in the Field that has Revolutionized*

Medicine, New York, NY, Kaplan Publishing, 2009.

O'Connor, Paul, *Multiple Sclerosis: The Facts You Need* (4th ed), Toronto, ON, Key Porter Books, 2009.

Ostalecki, Sharon, *Fibromyalgia: The Complete Guide from Medical Experts and Patients*, Sudbury, Massachusetts, Jones and Bartlett Publishers, 2008.

Podesto, Martine (Gen. Editor) et al, *Ultimate Canadian Medical Encyclopedia: Understanding, Preventing and Treating Medical Conditions*, Richmond Hill, Ontario, Firefly Books, 2010.

Potter, Steven, *Designer Genes: A New Era in the Evolution of Man*, New York, NY, Random House, 2010.

Ramachandran, V.S., *The Tell-Tale Brain: A Neuroscientist's Quest for What Makes Us Human*, New York, NY, WW Norton & Company, 2011.

Restak, Richard M., *Brainscapes: An Introduction to What Neuroscience has Learned About the Structure, Function, and Abilities of the Brain*, New York, NY, Hyperion/Discover, 1995.

Sharma, Nutan, Richman, Elaine, *Parkinson's Disease and the Family: A New Guide*, London, England, Harvard University Press, 2005.

Shenk, David, *The Forgetting: Alzheimer's: Portrait of an Epidemic*, Doubleday, New York, 2001.

Smiley, Jane, *The Man Who Invented the Computer: The Biography of John Atanasoff,* Toronto, Ontario, 2010.

Tosen, Paris, *American Androids Critical Edition*, Vancouver, BC, CreateSpace, 2013.

Tosen, Paris, *Reality Science*, Vancouver, BC, CreateSpace, 2013.

Tsiaras, Alexander, text by Werth, Barry, *The Architecture and Design of Man and Woman: The Marvel of the Human Body, Revealed,* New York, NY, Doubleday, 2004.

Venter, J. Craig, *A Life Decoded: My Genome: My Life*, London, England, Viking, 2007.

Watson, James D., w/Berry, Andrew, *DNA: The Secret of Life*, Alfred A. Knopf, New York/Toronto, 2003.

Wehr, Gerhard, Weeks, David M. (translator), *Jung, a Biography*, Shambhala, 1987.

White, Ruth C., Preston, John D., *Bipolar 101: A Practical Guide to Identifying Triggers, Managing Medications, Coping with Symptoms, and More*, Oakland, CA, New Harbinger Publications, 2009.

"That was in my eleventh year. There I— certainly—on my way to school, I stepped out of a mist. It was just as if I had been in a mist, walking in a mist, and stepped out of it and knew 'I am...I am what I am.' And then I thought, but what have I been before? And then I found that I had been in a mist. Not knowing to differentiate myself from things. I was just one thing, about, among many things."

~ Carl Jung

www.tosen.ca

www.ingramcontent.com/pod-product-compliance
Lightning Source LLC
Chambersburg PA
CBHW070850180526
45168CB00005B/1764